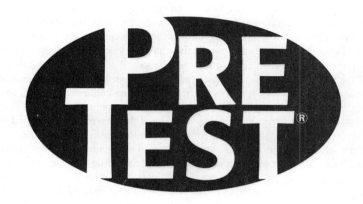

Obstetrics and Gynecology

PreTest® Self-Assessment and Review

NOTICE

Medicine is an ever-changing science. As new research and clinical experience broaden our knowledge, changes in treatment and drug therapy are required. The authors and the publisher of this work have checked with sources believed to be reliable in their efforts to provide information that is complete and generally in accord with the standards accepted at the time of publication. However, in view of the possibility of human error or changes in medical sciences, neither the authors nor the publisher nor any other party who has been involved in the preparation or publication of this work warrants that the information contained herein is in every respect accurate or complete, and they disclaim all responsibility for any errors or omissions or for the results obtained from use of the information contained in this work. Readers are encouraged to confirm the information contained herein with other sources. For example and in particular, readers are advised to check the product information sheet included in the package of each drug they plan to administer to be certain that the information contained in this work is accurate and that changes have not been made in the recommended dose or in the contraindications for administration. This recommendation is of particular importance in connection with new or infrequently used drugs.

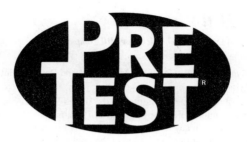

Obstetrics and Gynecology
PreTest® Self-Assessment and Review
Ninth Edition

MARK I. EVANS, M.D.

Professor and Chairman of Obstetrics and Gynecology
Professor of Human Genetics
Director, Fetal Therapy Program
MCP/Hahnemann University
Philadelphia, Pennsylvania

KENNETH A. GINSBURG, M.D.

Associate Professor
Department of Obstetrics and Gynecology
Director of Clinical Curriculum Development
Wayne State University School of Medicine
Detroit, Michigan

McGraw-Hill
Medical Publishing Division
PreTest® Series

NEW YORK   ST. LOUIS   SAN FRANCISCO   AUCKLAND
BOGOTÁ   CARACAS   LISBON   LONDON   MADRID
MEXICO CITY   MILAN   MONTREAL   NEW DELHI
SAN JUAN   SINGAPORE   SYDNEY   TOKYO   TORONTO

McGraw-Hill

*A Division of The **McGraw·Hill** Companies*

Obstetrics and Gynecology: PreTest Self-Assessment and Review, Ninth Edition
Copyright © 2001, 1998, 1995, 1992, 1989, 1987, 1985, 1982, 1978 by The **McGraw-Hill Companies, Inc.** All rights reserved. Printed in the United States of America. Except as permitted under the United States Copyright Act of 1976, no part of this publication may be reproduced or distributed in any form or by any means, or stored in a data base or retrieval system, without the prior written permission of the publisher.

5 6 7 8 9 0 DOC/DOC 0 9 8 7 6 5 4 3 2

ISBN 0-07-135961-3

This book was set in Berkeley by North Market Street Graphics.
The editor was Catherine Wenz.
The production supervisor was Minal Bopaiah.
Project management was provided by North Market Street Graphics.
The text designer was Jim Sullivan / RepCat Graphics & Editorial Services.
R.R. Donnelley & Sons was printer and binder.

This book is printed on acid-free paper.

Library of Congress Cataloging-in-Publication Data

Obstetrics and gynecology : PreTest self-assessment and review / edited by Mark I. Evans.—9th ed.
    p. ; cm.
    Includes bibliographical references.
    ISBN 0-07-135961-3
    1. Obstetrics—Examinations, questions, etc. 2. Gynecology—Examinations, questions, etc. I. Evans, Mark I.
  [DNLM: 1. Gynecology—Examination Questions. 2. Obstetrics—Examination Questions. WP 18.2 O14 2001]
RG111 .O37 2001
618'.076—dc21   00-060081

CONTENTS

OBSTETRICS

EARLY PREGNANCY

GENETICS, FETAL INFECTIONS, CONGENITAL ANOMALIES, PRENATAL DIAGNOSIS, AND ULTRASOUND

MEDICAL, SURGICAL, AND OBSTETRIC COMPLICATIONS OF PREGNANCY

ANTEPARTUM SURVEILLANCE, LABOR, AND DELIVERY

LACTATION, PUERPERIUM, AND BEHAVIORAL, ETHICAL, AND LEGAL PROBLEMS

GYNECOLOGY

ANATOMY, PUBERTY, MENSTRUATION, AND MENOPAUSE

PREFACE

No longer can students assume that continuing education ends with the completion of formal training and the successful completion of licensing or certifying examinations. As of October 1979, all 22 member boards of the American Board of Medical Specialties committed themselves to the principle of periodic recertification of their members. Despite the Board's recognition that the cognitive skills measured in the objective examination do not assure clinical competence, recertification efforts—insofar as they involve examinations—are based on the assumption that knowledge of current information on which good clinical decisions should be made is worth cultivating; that, while such information does not guarantee competent practice, lack of it probably impedes competent practice, that this knowledge, unlike technical skills, is reasonably easy to assess; and that it can be acquired by well-motivated physicians. These assumptions all seem reasonable.

The questions presented in this book deal with issues of relative importance to medical students; other problem-oriented materials are becoming available that are aimed at more sophisticated audiences— groups that, within a very few years, will include the present generation of students. Regular review of such material is a habit worth developing. We hope that this edition of *Obstetrics and Gynecology: PreTest® Self-Assessment and Review* will justify your efforts in working through the problems by providing guidance for further study and by helping you to develop enduring learning habits.

MARK I. EVANS, M.D.

KENNETH A. GINSBURG, M.D.

INTRODUCTION

Obstetrics and Gynecology: PreTest® Self-Assessment and Review, Ninth Edition, has been designed to provide medical students, as well as physicians, with a comprehensive and convenient instrument for self-assessment and review within the field of obstetrics and gynecology. The 500 questions provided have been designed to parallel the format of the questions contained in Step 2 of the United States Medical Licensing Examination (USMLE).

Each question in the book is accompanied by an answer, a paragraph explanation, and a specific page reference to a current textbook. A bibliography that lists all the sources used in the book follows the last chapter.

Perhaps the most effective way to use this book is to allow yourself one minute to answer each question in a given chapter; as you proceed, indicate your answer beside each question. By following this suggestion, you will be approximating the time limits imposed by licensing examinations.

When you practice your examination-taking skills with this PreTest®, one way to maximize your score is to go through, answer all the questions you find easy, and skip over the more difficult ones initially. We do recommend, however, that once you come back to the more difficult questions, you spend as much time as you need. You will then be more likely to retain the information.

When you have finished answering the questions in a chapter, you should then spend as much time as you need verifying your answers and carefully reading the explanations. Although you should pay special attention to the explanations for the questions you answered incorrectly, you should read every explanation. The authors of this book have designed the explanations to reinforce and supplement the information tested by the questions. If, after reading the explanations for a given chapter, you feel you need still more information about the material covered, you may wish to consult the references indicated.

OBSTETRICS

EARLY PREGNANCY

Questions

DIRECTIONS: Each item below contains a question or incomplete statement followed by suggested responses. Select the **one best** response to each question.

1. Maternal mortality refers to the number of maternal deaths that occur as the result of the reproductive process per

a. 1000 births
b. 10,000 births
c. 100,000 births
d. 10,000 live births
e. 100,000 live births

2. The most common cause of maternal death in the United States is

a. Abortion
b. Anesthesia
c. Embolism
d. Ectopic pregnancy
e. Hemorrhage

3. Which of the following is included in the fertility rate?

a. Women age 14 years
b. 400-g fetuses
c. Births per 1000 population
d. Births per 1000 females age 15 to 45 years
e. Stillbirths

4. Which of the following statements about twinning is true?

a. The frequencies of monozygosity and dizygosity are the same
b. Division after formation of the embryonic disk results in conjoined twins
c. The incidence of monozygotic twinning varies with race
d. A dichorionic twin pregnancy always denotes dizygosity
e. Twinning causes no appreciable increase in maternal morbidity and mortality over singleton pregnancies

DIRECTIONS: Each group of questions below consists of lettered options followed by numbered items. For each numbered item, select the appropriate lettered option(s). Each lettered option may be used once, more than once, or not at all. **Choose exactly the number of options indicated following each item.**

Items 5–9

Match each description with the correct type of abortion.

a. Complete abortion
b. Incomplete abortion
c. Threatened abortion
d. Missed abortion
e. Inevitable abortion

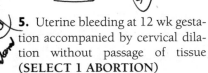

5. Uterine bleeding at 12 wk gestation accompanied by cervical dilation without passage of tissue **(SELECT 1 ABORTION)**

6. Passage of some but not all placental tissue through the cervix at 9 wk gestation **(SELECT 1 ABORTION)**

7. Fetal death at 15 wk gestation without expulsion of any fetal or maternal tissue for at least 8 wk **(SELECT 1 ABORTION)**

8. Uterine bleeding at 7 wk gestation without any cervical dilation **(SELECT 1 ABORTION)**

9. Expulsion of all fetal and placental tissue from the uterine cavity at 10 wk gestation **(SELECT 1 ABORTION)**

10. Components of sperm capacitation include

a. Cyclic guanosine 5′-monophosphate (GMP) formation
b. Decreased permeability to calcium
c. Maintenance of a high intracellular calcium concentration
d. Maintenance of a low potassium concentration
e. Acrosome reaction

11. True statements about human chorionic gonadotropin (hCG) include

a. It is produced by the cytotrophoblast
b. It is a glycoprotein
c. Levels peak at the midpoint of pregnancy
d. It is composed of four subunits
e. It is low in carbohydrate content

12. The placenta of twins may be

a. Dichorionic and monoamniotic in dizygotic (DZ) twins
b. Dichorionic and monoamniotic in monozygotic (MZ) twins
c. Monochorionic and monoamniotic in DZ twins
d. Dichorionic and diamniotic in MZ twins

13. The most important factor in the regulation of placental transfer of glutamine is which of the following?

a. The metabolism by the fetus during transfer
b. The area for exchange within the fetal arteries
c. The bound concentration of the substance in the fetal blood
d. The specific binding or carrier proteins in the fetal or maternal circulation
e. A positive transfer gradient from the mother to the fetus

14. In the embryologic development of the human kidney

a. The pronephros has no ultimate function
b. The mesonephros replaces the pronephros in the 10th wk
c. The metanephros forms lower in the cavity than the original kidney
d. The müllerian duct originates during the 12th wk
e. The müllerian duct develops at the same time as the pronephros

15. Compared with its adult weight, the fetal organ that is the largest is the

a. Heart
b. Thymus
c. Gallbladder
d. Adrenal cortex
e. Stomach

16. Fetal blood is returned to the umbilical arteries and the placenta through the

a. Hypogastric arteries
b. Ductus venosus
c. Portal vein
d. Inferior vena cava
e. Foramen ovale

17. A primitive fetal circulation is established how many days after ovulation?

a. 7
b. 14
c. 21
d. 28
e. 35

18. True statements regarding embryonic implantation include which of the following?

a. It occurs when the embryo first reaches the endometrial cavity
b. It is prevented by the birth control pill
c. It requires the removal of the zona pellucida
d. The fetomaternal circulation is first established by the invasion of spiral arteries
e. The uteroplacental circulation is established 7 days after ovulation

19. The finding of a single umbilical artery on examination of the umbilical cord after delivery is

a. Insignificant
b. Equal in incidence in blacks and whites
c. An indicator of considerably increased incidence of major malformation of the fetus
d. Equally common in newborns of diabetic and nondiabetic mothers
e. Present in 5% of all births

Items 20–24

For each structure below, select its embryologic origin.

a. Genital tubercle
b. Genital swellings
c. Urogenital sinus
d. Urethral folds
e. Müllerian ducts

20. Labia minora (**SELECT 1 ORIGIN**)

21. Labia majora (**SELECT 1 ORIGIN**)

22. Clitoris (**SELECT 1 ORIGIN**)

23. Lower one-third of vagina (**SELECT 1 ORIGIN**)

24. Fallopian tubes (**SELECT 1 ORIGIN**)

25. After an initial pregnancy resulted in a spontaneous loss in the first trimester, your patient is concerned about the possibility of this recurring. An appropriate answer would be that the chance of recurrence

a. Depends on the genetic makeup of the prior abortus
b. Is no different than it was prior to the miscarriage
c. Is increased to approximately 50%
d. Is increased most likely to greater than 50%
e. Depends on the sex of the prior abortus

26. A 24-year-old woman has had three first-trimester spontaneous abortions. Which of the following statements concerning chromosomal aberrations in abortions is true?

a. 45,X is more prevalent in chromosomally abnormal term babies than in abortus products
b. Approximately 20% of first-trimester spontaneous abortions have chromosomal abnormalities
c. Trisomy 21 is the most common trisomy in abortuses
d. Despite the relatively high frequency of Down syndrome at term, most Down fetuses abort spontaneously
e. Stillbirths have twice the incidence of chromosomal abnormalities as live births

27. Rates of successful pregnancy following three spontaneous losses (habitual abortion) are

a. Very poor
b. Slightly worse than those in the baseline population
c. No different from those in the baseline population
d. Just under 50%
e. Good unless cervical incompetence is diagnosed

28. A 26-year-old patient has had three consecutive spontaneous abortions early in the second trimester. As part of an evaluation for this problem, the least useful test would be

a. Hysterosalpingogram
b. Chromosomal analysis of the couple
c. Endometrial biopsy in the luteal phase
d. Postcoital test
e. Tests of thyroid function

Items 29–30

A 19-year-old primigravid woman is expecting her first child; she is 12 wk pregnant by dates. She has vaginal bleeding and an enlarged-for-dates uterus. In addition, no fetal heart sounds are heard. The ultrasound below is obtained.

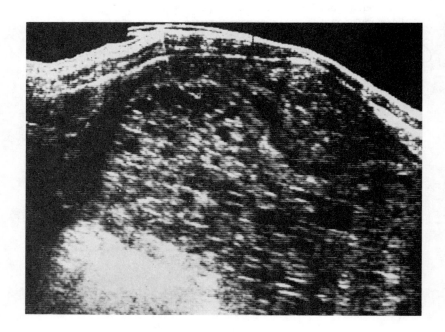

29. The most likely diagnosis of this woman's condition is

a. Sarcoma botryoides
b. Tuberculous endometritis
c. Adenocarcinoma of the uterus
d. Hydatidiform mole
e. Normal pregnancy

30. After uterine evacuation, management of the woman described above, who has no clinical or radiographic evidence of metastatic disease, should include

a. Weekly hCG titers
b. Hysterectomy
c. Single-agent chemotherapy
d. Combination chemotherapy
e. Radiation therapy

31. Which of the statements regarding the karyotype shown below is true?

a. There are six group E chromosomes
b. The phenotype is female
c. The extra chromosome is acrocentric
d. The chance of a cardiac anomaly is approximately 10%
e. The origin of the extra chromosome is likely paternal

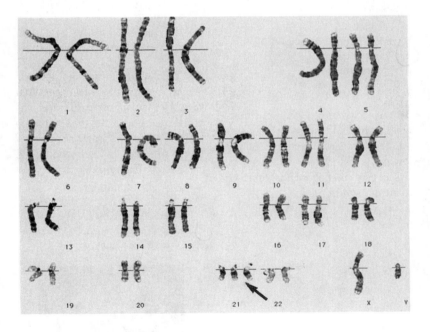

32. The risk of having a baby with Down syndrome for a 30-year-old woman increases

a. If the father of the baby is age 40
b. If her pregnancy has been achieved by induction of ovulation by menotropins (e.g. Follistin, Gonal F)
c. If she has had a previous baby with Turner syndrome (45,X)
d. If she has had a previous baby with triploidy
e. If she has had three first-trimester spontaneous abortions

33. In terms of birth defect potential, the safest of the following drugs is

a. Alcohol
b. Isotretinoin (Accutane)
c. Tetracyclines
d. Progesterones
e. Phenytoin (Dilantin)

34. A 15-year-old has primary amenorrhea and no secondary sexual development. Which of the following is associated with gonadal dysgenesis phenotype (as opposed to Turner syndrome)?

a. 45,X
b. 46,XXr
c. 46,XXp−
d. 46,Xi(Xq)
e. 46,X,i(Xp)

35. A carrier of a balanced 14/21 (D/G) translocation is described by which of the following statements?

a. Amniocentesis, but not chorionic villus sampling, can detect offspring who have translocation Down syndrome as well as those who are balanced carriers
b. Karyotype analysis would reveal 46 chromosomes in each cell
c. Chromosome studies of members of a carrier's family are indicated to detect others at risk for having children with Down syndrome
d. The risk for bearing children who have Down syndrome is the same whether the husband or the wife is the carrier
e. The risk of an unbalanced translocation increases with maternal age

36. A 32-year-old woman, gravida 3, para 3, presents with abdominal pain. Her last menstrual period was 6 wk ago, and a pregnancy test is positive. The specimen shown below is obtained at laparotomy. The most likely diagnosis is

a. Incomplete abortion
b. Missed abortion
c. Hydatidiform mole
d. Tubal ectopic pregnancy
e. Ovarian pregnancy

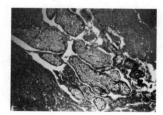

37. A 19-year-old woman comes to the emergency room and reports that she fainted at work earlier in the day. She has mild vaginal bleeding. Her abdomen is diffusely tender and distended. In addition, she complains of shoulder and abdominal pain. Her temperature is 36.4°C (97.6°F), pulse rate is 120 beats/min, and blood pressure is 96/50 mm Hg. To confirm the diagnosis suggested by the available clinical data, the best diagnostic procedure would be

a. Pregnancy test
b. Posterior colpotomy
c. Dilation and curettage
d. Culdocentesis
e. Laparoscopy

38. Women at increased risk for the development of gestational trophoblastic disease include those

a. With sickle cell trait
b. In South America
c. Under 30 years of age
d. Who are strict vegetarians
e. With vitamin C deficiency

39. Which of the following is most reliably associated with molar pregnancy?

a. Urinary incontinence
b. Fecal incontinence
c. Preeclampsia in early pregnancy
d. Hyperemesis gravidarum
e. Threatened abortion

40. In patients with small ectopic pregnancies, medical management may include

a. Actinomycin D
b. RU-486 (progesterone antagonist)
c. Prostaglandin $F_{2\alpha}$
d. Methotrexate
e. Isotretinoin

41. Indications for instituting single-agent chemotherapy following evacuation of a hydatidiform mole usually include

a. A rise in hCG titers
b. A plateau of hCG titers for 1 wk
c. Return of hCG titers to normal at 6 wk after evacuation
d. Appearance of liver metastases
e. Appearance of brain metastases

42. Observations on the role of actinomycin D and methotrexate in the management of gestational trophoblastic disease suggest that

a. Resistance to one agent results in cross-resistance to the other
b. Methotrexate is safer than actinomycin D for women whose liver function is impaired
c. There is no additive effect in combining the two agents
d. Actinomycin D is as effective as methotrexate for primary treatment
e. Alkylating agents are an alternative to methotrexate for single-agent therapy

43. In comparing laparoscopic salpingostomy versus laparotomy with salpingectomy for the treatment of ectopic pregnancies, laparoscopic therapy results in

a. Decreased hospital stays
b. A lower fertility rate
c. A lower repeat ectopic pregnancy rate
d. A comparable persistent ectopic tissue rate
e. Greater scar formation

44. Velamentous insertion of cord is associated with increased risk for

a. Premature rupture of membranes
b. Fetal exsanguination before labor
c. Torsion of the umbilical cord
d. Fetal malformations
e. Uterine malformations

45. A 27-year-old has just had an ectopic pregnancy. Which of these preceeding events would be most likely to predispose to this ectopic?

a. Previous tubal surgery
b. Pelvic inflammatory disease (PID)
c. Use of a contraceptive intrauterine device (IUD)
d. Induction of ovulation
e. Exposure in utero to diethylstilbestrol (DES)

46. Chorioangiomas can be described by which of the following statements?

a. They affect more than 5% of placentas
b. They are often associated with anomalous cord insertions
c. They are often associated with cords containing only two vessels
d. They are the most common tumors of the placenta
e. They are associated with trisomy 18 fetuses

47. Signs helpful in pointing toward pelvic infection in differentiating it from a tubal pregnancy include which of the following?

a. High fever
b. Enlarged uterus
c. Presence of β-hCG
d. Leukocytosis
e. Nausea

48. Nausea and vomiting are common in pregnancy. Hyperemesis gravidarum, however, is a much more serious and potentially fatal problem. Findings that should alert the physician to the diagnosis of hyperemesis gravidarum early in its course include

a. Electrocardiographic evidence of hypokalemia
b. Metabolic acidosis
c. Jaundice
d. Ketonuria

49. A 24-year-old woman is in a car accident and is taken to an emergency room, where she receives a chest x-ray and film of her lower spine. It is later discovered that she is 10 wk pregnant. She should be counseled that

a. The fetus has received 50 rads
b. Either chorionic villus sampling (CVS) or amniocentesis is advisable to check for fetal chromosomal abnormalities
c. At 10 wk the fetus is particularly susceptible to derangements of the central nervous system
d. The fetus has received rads below the assumed threshold for radiation damage
e. The risk that this fetus will develop leukemia as a child is raised

Items 50–52

A 47-year-old woman has achieved a pregnancy with in vitro fertilization (IVF) using donor eggs from a 21-year-old donor and sperm from her 46-year-old husband. Four embryos were transferred; the patient has a quintuplet pregnancy at 10 wk gestation.

50. The above patient wants to know what is the chance that at least one of the embryos has a chromosome abnormality. The risk for a singleton pregnancy at term for a 47-year-old is 1 in 7, and for a 21-year-old is 1 in 550.

a. 1/7
b. 4/7
c. 5/7
d. 4/550
e. 5/550

51. The patient is considering undergoing selective fetal reduction. True statements include

a. The procedure cannot be done with quintuplets
b. Risks for the procedure are greater than the risks of carrying the quintuplets
c. Procedure risk rates are comparable among all practitioners
d. α fetoprotein is a useful marker for Down syndrome after the procedure
e. The risk of prematurity, as well as loss, will be lowered by reduction

52. On ultrasound prior to the procedure, a 5-mm nuchal translucency is discovered in one of the embryos. Implications of this finding include

a. The embryo has a high risk of neural tube defect
b. The embryo has a high risk of a cardiac malformation
c. The nuchal translucency will enlarge by 20 wk
d. If the nuchal translucency resolves, the risk of a chromosome abnormality is comparable to that of other embryos
e. If aneuploid, the most likely diagnosis is Turner syndrome

EARLY PREGNANCY

Answers

1. The answer is e. *(Gleicher, 3/e, p 17. Heppard, 2/e, p 378. Scott, 8/e, p 90.)* Maternal mortality is a ratio, not a rate, and is calculated per 100,000 live births. Although there have been marked advances in prenatal care associated with a declining maternal mortality over the past 25 years, there still exist subgroups of the female population at much higher risk. These include black women (apparently because of social and economic conditions), women of high parity, and the older gravida. About 50% of maternal deaths in the United States are caused by hemorrhage, hypertension, or infection.

2. The answer is c. *(Heppard, 2/e, p 378. Gleicher, 3/e, p 17.)* Maternal mortality in the United States has fallen dramatically over the past 50 years. In 1935 the rate was approximately 582 deaths per 100,000 live births. By 1985 it had fallen to 7.8 per 100,000 live births, or approximately 1 per 12,820 live births. Death from ectopic pregnancy would be counted in the numerator, but not the denominator. The most common cause of death is embolism, constituting 17% of the total. Hypertension accounts for 12%, ectopic pregnancy 10%, hemorrhage 9%, stroke 8%, anesthesia 7%, abortion-related causes 5%, cardiomyopathy 4%, infection 3.5%, and indirect causes 16%. In other parts of the world, mortality is still much higher and the percentages are different.

3. The answer is d. *(Scott, 8/e, p 90.)* The birth rate is the number of live births per 1000 population, and by definition includes males and females. The fertility rate is the number of live births per 1000 females ages 15 to 44 years. For a fetus to be counted as a delivery, it must have reached 500 g. Both birth and fertility rates refer to live births; therefore, stillbirths are excluded.

4. The answer is b. *(Gall, pp 1–3, 24–27.)* The incidence of monozygotic twinning is constant at a rate of one set per 250 births around the world. It is unaffected by race, heredity, age, parity, or infertility agents. Examination of the amnion and chorion can be used to determine monozygosity only if one chorion is identified. Two identifiable chorions can occur in monozygotic or dizygotic twinning. The time of the division of a fertilized zygote to form monozygotic twins determines the placental and membranous anatomy. Late division after formation of the embryonic disk will result in conjoined twins.

5–9. The answers are 5-e, 6-b, 7-d, 8-c, 9-a. *(Scott, 8/e, pp 143–146.)* Bleeding occurs in about 30% to 40% of human gestations before 20 wk of pregnancy, with about half of these pregnancies ending in spontaneous abortion. A threatened abortion takes place when this uterine bleeding occurs without any cervical dilation or effacement.

In a patient bleeding during the first half of pregnancy, the diagnosis of inevitable abortion is strengthened if the bleeding is profuse and associated with uterine cramping pains. If cervical dilation has occurred, with or without rupture of membranes, the abortion is inevitable.

If only a portion of the products of conception has been expelled and the cervix remains dilated, a diagnosis of incomplete abortion is made. However, if all fetal and placental tissue has been expelled, the cervix is closed, bleeding from the canal is minimal or decreasing, and uterine cramps have ceased, a diagnosis of complete abortion can be made.

The diagnosis of missed abortion is suspected when the uterus fails to continue to enlarge with or without uterine bleeding or spotting. A missed abortion is one in which fetal death occurs before 20 wk gestation without expulsion of any fetal or maternal tissue for at least 8 wk thereafter. When a fetus is retained in the uterus beyond 5 wk after fetal death, consumptive coagulability with hypofibrogenemia may occur. This is uncommon, however, in gestations of less than 14 wk duration.

10. The answer is e. *(Speroff, 6/e, pp 251–252.)* Capacitation is a multistep process beginning with initial exposure post ejaculation to seminal plasma. Motility results as a function of increased adenylate cyclase and cyclic adenosine 5′-monophosphate (AMP)-dependent kinase systems. Increased adenyl cyclase activity requires calcium for capacitation. The spermatozoa maintain an environment characterized by high intracellular potassium, low sodium, and low calcium, which is maintained by a potassium/sodium pump.

11. The answer is b. (*Speroff, 6/e, pp 291–296.*) hCG is a glycoprotein with a high carbohydrate content. It is a heterodimer with two dissimilar units designated α and β, which are noncovalently linked. The syncytiotrophoblast, not the cytotrophoblast, produces hCG, and the dissociated free β is the active component. Levels rise dramatically throughout the first trimester, peaking at approximately 12 wk, and then fall rapidly. The rate of rise of hCG in the first trimester can be used to define gestational age and to assess the adequacy of implantation, e.g., vis-à-vis ectopic and threatened abortions.

12. The answer is d. (*Gall, pp 1–3, 25–26.*) Dizygotic twins of different sexes always have a dichorionic and diamniotic placenta and monochorionic monozygotic twins are always of the same sex. The dichorionic placentas of dizygotic twins may be totally separated or intimately fused. Of monozygotic twins, 20% to 30% have dichorionic placentation, the result of separation of the blastocyst in the first 2 days after fertilization. The majority of monozygotic twins have a diamniotic and monochorionic placenta. The least common type of placentation in monozygotic twins is the monochorionic and monoamniotic placenta; its incidence is only about 1%.

13. The answer is d. (*Reece, 2/e, p 1061–1062.*) There are multiple variables that are important in determining the effectiveness of the placenta in transferring nutrients. Concentration gradients, specific transport mechanisms, and the integrity of the placental unit are factors in determining the rate and amount of transfer. For example, there is a net transfer of all amino acids from the mother to the fetus, except for glutamine, which is used to transfer excess nitrogen amino groups back to the mother.

14. The answer is a. (*DiSaia, 5/e, p 36.*) The first kidney, the pronephros, does not seem to have any human function and is replaced by the mesonephros in approximately the 4th wk. The mesonephros has tubules similar to those of its predecessor. The definitive kidney, the metanephros, supplants the mesonephros beginning in the 6th or 7th wk. Its duct originates as an outpouching of the lower end of the mesonephros, which then grows upward. The müllerian duct originates during approximately the 6th wk and degenerates in males at approximately the 10th wk.

15. The answer is d. *(Reece, 2/e, p 95.)* The fetal adrenal cortex is the largest organ of the fetus, having as much as 85% of the weight of the adult adrenal cortex. The structure of the cortex, however, is somewhat different in that there is a fetal zone that disappears in the adult adrenal. The other organs, while proportionally larger in the term fetus than in the adult, are not nearly as large. Compared with the adult adrenal, the fetal adrenal cortex synthesizes large amounts of pregnenolone sulfate and dehydroepiandrosterone sulfate, and only a small amount of cortisol.

16. The answer is a. *(Reece, 2/e, pp 54, 119–121.)* Fetal blood is returned directly to the placenta through the two hypogastric arteries. The distal portions of the hypogastric arteries atrophy and obliterate within 3 to 4 days after birth; remnants are called umbilical ligaments. Fetal oxygenation is aided by the presence of three vascular shunts: ductus venosus, foramen ovale, and ductus arteriosus. The ductus venosus shunts oxygenated blood from the umbilical vein into the inferior vena cava. The foramen ovale deflects the more oxygenated blood from the right atrium into the left atrium, thereby bypassing pulmonary circulation. Approximately two-thirds of the blood ejected from the right ventricle is shunted away from pulmonary circulation through the ductus arteriosus.

17. The answer is c. *(Reece, 2/e, pp 29–43.)* Angiogenesis can be seen in the extraembryonic mesoderm of the yolk sac by day 15 or 16 post ovulation. Primitive blood cells develop from endothelial cells 2 to 3 days later, as the vessels develop on the yolk sac and allantois. Separate mesenchymal cells surrounding the endothelial vessels differentiate into muscular and connective tissue elements. The primitive heart forms from mesenchymal cells in a similar manner in the cardiogenic area. Paired endothelial channels called heart tubes develop by the end of the 3rd wk and fuse to form the primitive heart. By the 21st day, the primitive heart has linked up with blood vessels to form a primitive embryonic cardiovascular system. Blood circulation starts about this time and the cardiovascular system becomes the first functioning organ system in the embryo.

18. The answer is c. *(Scott, 8/e, p 30.)* The embryo reaches the endometrial cavity 3 days after ovulation, at the morula–early blastocyst stage. The birth control pill prevents ovulation but does not affect implantation. Implantation starts about 3 days later, following removal of the zona pellucida on day 4 to

5 (post ovulation). On day 7 to 8, the trophoblast differentiates into cytotrophoblast and syncytiotrophoblast. The endometrial capillaries in contact with the invading syncytiotrophoblast coalesce to form venous sinuses. Endometrial spiral arteries are not invaded at this point. The trophoblast invades endometrial sinusoids, establishing a uteroplacental circulation by 11 to 12 days post ovulation. A day later, the endometrium completely covers the blastocyst.

19. The answer is c. (*Jaffe, pp 96–97.*) The absence of one umbilical artery occurs in 0.7% to 0.8% of all umbilical cords of singletons, in 2.5% of all abortuses, and in approximately 5% of at least one twin. The incidence of a single artery is significantly increased in newborns of diabetic mothers, and it occurs in white infants twice as often as in newborns of black women. The incidence of major fetal malformations when only one artery is identified has been reported to be as high as 18% and there is an increased incidence of overall fetal mortality. The finding is an indication to offer amniocentesis, cordocentesis, or chorionic villus sampling to study fetal chromosomes, although there is debate when there is only a truly isolated finding of single umbilical artery.

20–24. The answers are 20-d, 21-b, 22-a, 23-c, 24-e. (*Gidwani, pp 9–11. Rock, 8/e, pp 63–64.*) In the female, the urethral folds give rise to the labia minora, while the labia majora are formed from the genital swellings. It is believed that the development of external genitalia is dependent on the presence of hormones during the intrauterine period. With the absence of androgens and the inducer substance in females, the wolffian duct system regresses while the external genitalia develop under the influence of estrogen from both maternal and placental sources.

In the male, the genital tubercle gives rise to the phallus, while in the female it elongates minimally to form the clitoris. Clitoral hypertrophy can occur in conditions under which there is an abnormally high level of circulating androgens during the critical phase of development of the external genitalia. Congenital adrenal hyperplasia and mixed gonadal dysgenesis are two clinical situations that may present with clitoral hypertrophy.

There are several theories to explain the embryologic origin of the vagina; however, it is generally accepted that the upper two-thirds of the vagina are of müllerian duct origin while the lower one-third is of urogenital sinus origin, which seems to explain in part the congenital anomalies that arise in this anatomic region. A common anomaly of urogenital sinus origin is imperforate hymen, which is easily treated by hymenotomy. Congenital absence of the vagina is an anomaly of müllerian duct origin and, as such, usually involves an absence of only the upper two-thirds of the vagina, as well as an absence of the uterus and fallopian tubes in most cases.

In the female, the müllerian ducts give rise to the fallopian tubes, uterus, and cervix. Imperfect fusion of the müllerian ducts can give rise to a whole spectrum of uterine anomalies, which may be associated with clinical entities such as habitual abortions, prematurity, and fetal malpositions. Patients with proven müllerian duct anomalies should have an intravenous pyelogram to rule out urinary tract anomalies that may be present.

25. The answer is b. (*Adashi, pp 2245–2255.*) An initial spontaneous abortion, irrespective of the karyotype or sex of the child, does not change the risk for having a recurrence in a future pregnancy. The rate is commonly quoted as 15% of all known pregnancies.

26. The answer is d. (*Keye, pp 230–245. Speroff, 6/e, p 1045.*) Chromosomal abnormalities are found in approximately 50% of spontaneous abortions, 5% of stillbirths, and 0.5% of live born babies. In the spontaneous losses, trisomy 16 is the most common trisomy, with 45,X the most common single abnormality found. At term, trisomy 16 is never seen and 45,X is seen in approximately 1 in 2,000 births. It is estimated that 99% of 45,X and 75% of trisomy 21 conceptuses are lost before term.

27. The answer is b. (*Adashi, pp 2245–2255.*) A variety of therapies have resulted in successful pregnancy rates of 70% to 85% following a diagnosis of habitual abortion. When cervical incompetence is present and a cerclage is placed, success rates range as high as 90%.

28. The answer is d. (*Fleisher, 5/e, pp 732–735. Ransom 2000, pp 511–515.*) The history, clinical picture, and ultrasound of the woman described in the question are characteristic of hydatidiform mole. The most common initial symptoms include an enlarged-for-dates uterus and continuous or intermittent bleeding in the first two trimesters. Other symptoms include hypertension, proteinuria, and hyperthyroidism. Hydatidiform mole is 10 times as common in the Far East as in North America, and it occurs more frequently in women over 45 years of age. A tissue sample would show a villus with hydropic changes and no vessels. Grossly, these lesions appear as small, clear clusters of grapelike vesicles, the passage of which confirms the diagnosis.

29. The answer is a. *(Rock, 8/e, pp 1631–1632.)* The condition of women who have hydatidiform moles but no evidence of metastatic disease should be followed routinely by hCG titers after uterine evacuation. Most authorities agree that prophylactic chemotherapy should not be employed in the routine management of women having hydatidiform moles because 85% to 90% of affected patients will require no further treatment. For a young woman in whom preservation of reproductive function is important, surgery is not routinely indicated.

30. The answer is d. *(Speroff, 6/e, 1043–1052.)* A major cause of spontaneous abortions in the first trimester is chromosomal abnormalities; however, the causes of losses in the second trimester are more likely to be uterine or environmental in origin. Patients should be screened for thyroid function, diabetes mellitus, and collagen vascular disorders. There is also a correlation between patients with a positive lupus anticoagulant and recurrent miscarriages. A hysterosalpingogram should be performed to rule out uterine structural abnormalities, such as bicornuate uterus, septate uterus, unicornuate uterus, submucous fibroids, or intrauterine adhesions. Endometrial biopsy is performed to rule out an insufficiency of the luteal phase or evidence of chronic endometritis. If no abnormalities are found, both the husband and wife should be karyotyped to see if a balanced translocation or 45,X mosaicism exists. A postcoital test is useful for couples who cannot conceive but does not address postconception losses.

31. The answer is e. *(Rodeck, pp 437–438.)* Before banding techniques to discern the internal structures of chromosomes were available, chromosomes could only be put into groups by size and location of the centromere (A = 1, 2, 3; B = 4, 5; C = 6–12 and X; D = 13–15; E = 16–18; F = 19, 20; G = 21, 22, and Y). One X and one Y chromosome are seen (lower right) and indicate a male phenotype. A third chromosome 21 is seen consistent with Down syndrome, with which 50% of newborns have significant cardiac pathology. In the vast majority of cases, the nondisjunctional event is maternal.

32. The answer is e. *(Gleicher, 3/e, pp 173–178.)* The risk of aneuploidy is increased with multiple miscarriages not attributable to other causes such as endocrine abnormalities or cervical incompetence. Paternal age does not contribute significantly to aneuploidy until probably age 55, and most risks of paternal age are for point mutations. A 45,X karyotype results from loss of chromosome material and does not involve increased risks for nondisjunctional errors. Similarly, induced ovulation does not result in increased nondisjunction, and hypermodel conceptions (triploidy) do not increase risk for future pregnancies.

33. The answer is d. *(Gleicher, 3/e, pp 263–267.)* Alcohol is an enormous contributor to otherwise preventable birth defects. Sequelae include retardation of intrauterine growth, craniofacial abnormalities, and mental retardation. The occasional drink in pregnancy has not been proved to be deleterious. Isotretinoin (Accutane) is a powerful drug for acne that has enormous potential for producing congenital anomalies when ingested in early pregnancy; it should never be used in pregnancy. Tetracyclines interfere with development of bone and can lead to stained teeth in children. Progesterones have been implicated in multiple birth defects but controlled studies have failed to demonstrate a significant association with increased risk. Patients who have inadvertently become pregnant while on birth control pills should be reassured that the incidence of birth defects is no higher for them than for the general population. Phenytoin (Dilantin) is used for epilepsy and can be associated with a spectrum of abnormalities, including digital hypoplasia and facial abnormalities.

34. The answer is e. *(Remoin, 3/e, pp 971–980.)* Although monosomy of the X chromosome (45,X) is the most common karyotype of patients who have Turner syndrome, a variety of structural abnormalities of the X chromosome in addition to mosaics may be found in patients who have this disorder. Comparison of chromosomal abnormalities and phenotypic features in persons who have gonadal dysgenesis indicates that the short stature and other clinical findings of Turner phenotype are associated with loss of the short arm of one X chromosome. Of the karyotypes listed in the question, all involve monosomy for a portion of the short arm of the X chromosome except 46,X,i(Xp). People who have this karyotype have only one normal X chromosome; their other X chromosome, composed of a duplication of the normal short arm, is called an isochromosome. In essence, they are monosomic for the long arm of the X and trisomic for the short arm. This karyotype is associated with gonadal dysgenesis but not with the phenotypic features characteristic of persons who have Turner syndrome.

35. The answer is c. *(Gleicher, 3/e, pp 123–130.)* Persons who are carriers of a balanced D/G translocation have 45 chromosomes in each cell; one D-group and one G-group chromosome have fused, forming a chromosome that resembles a member of the C group. The risk for giving birth to children who have translocation Down syndrome is substantially higher if the wife is the carrier (10% to 12%) than if the husband is the carrier (2% to 3%) but does not change with age. Amniocentesis or CVS can determine whether the offspring will be unaffected, will carry the translocation, or will have the disease. Because a D/G translocation can be inherited from a parent (approximately 50% are familial), chromosomal studies of family members are recommended.

36. The answer is d. *(Scott, 8/e, pp 155–168.)* The photomicrograph accompanying the question shows villi within a tubular structure; the villi are easily identified by the presence of cytotrophoblasts. The diagnosis is tubal ectopic pregnancy. Molar pregnancy, incomplete abortion, and missed abortion also can be associated with the presence of villi, but specimens from these disorders would not be obtained at laparotomy.

37. The answer is d. *(Rock, 8/e, pp 121–122.)* The clinical history presented in this question is a classic one for a ruptured tubal pregnancy accompanied by hemoperitoneum. Because pregnancy tests are negative in almost 50% of cases, they are of little practical value in an emergency. Dilation and curettage would not permit rapid enough diagnosis, and the results obtained by this procedure are variable. Posterior colpotomy requires an operating room, surgical anesthesia, and an experienced operator with a scrubbed and gowned associate. Refined optic and electronic systems have improved the accuracy of laparoscopy, but this new equipment is not always available, and the procedure requires an operating room and, usually, surgical anesthesia. Culdocentesis is a rapid, nonsurgical method to confirm the presence of unclotted intraabdominal blood from a ruptured tubal pregnancy. Culdocentesis, however, is also not perfect, and a negative culdocentesis should not be used as the sole criteria for whether or not to operate on a patient.

38. The answer is d. (*Mishell, 3/e, pp 34–35, 997–998.*) Hydatidiform moles are seen in the United States in 1 of 1200 pregnancies. In the Far East rates as high as 1 in 77 pregnancies have been reported. Both younger and older patients appear to be at increased risk. It has been suggested that vitamin A deficiency and deficiencies of animal fat may be responsible for the higher incidence. Risk for recurrent trophoblastic disease has been reported as high as 1 in 50.

39. The answer is c. (*Rock, 8/e, pp 1631–1632.*) Early abortion frequently occurs in molar pregnancy. Uterine bleeding is the single outstanding sign, but is associated with many causes; it may vary from spotting to profuse hemorrhage. Although bleeding may appear only immediately prior to abortion, more often it occurs intermittently for weeks or even months preceding abortion. Toxemia of pregnancy, occurring early rather than in the third trimester as is expected in normal pregnancy, is seen in 10% to 15% of patients with molar pregnancy and suggests molar pregnancy until proven otherwise. Hyperemesis is a frequent complaint and is likely to be more severe and protracted in cases of molar pregnancy than in normal gestation. Urinary and fecal incontinence are rare and unrelated to molar pregnancy.

40. The answer is d. (*Mishell, 3/e, pp 455–457.*) Medical therapy for the management of ectopic pregnancies is still experimental, although it has been widely reported. The most common chemotherapeutic agent used at this time is methotrexate, a folic acid antagonist. Progesterone antagonists have not been successful in the management of ectopic pregnancies. Oral isotretinoin (Accutane), a powerful acne drug, is teratogenic and should never be used in pregnancy.

41. The answer is a. (*Mishell, 3/e, pp 455–456.*) Single-agent chemotherapy usually is instituted if levels of hCG have remained elevated 8 wk after evacuation of a hydatidiform mole. Approximately 50% of the patients who have persistently high hCG titers will develop malignant sequelae. If hCG titers rise or reach a plateau for 2 to 3 successive weeks following molar evacuation, a single-agent chemotherapy should be instituted, provided that the trophoblastic disease has not metastasized to the liver or brain. The presence of such metastases usually requires initiation of combination chemotherapy.

42. The answer is d. (*Mishell, 3/e, pp 455–458.*) The first successful treatment regimen for women with gestational trophoblastic disease consisted of single-agent methotrexate chemotherapy. Subsequent studies combining methotrexate, actinomycin D, and an alkylating agent were successful in treating methotrexate-resistant trophoblastic disease. Actinomycin D, then studied as a single agent, proved to be as effective as methotrexate; in addition, it was not hampered by cross-resistance in methotrexate-resistant tumors and was safer to use in women with impaired liver function.

43. The answer is a. (*Speroff, 6/e, p 1163.*) Conservative laparoscopic treatment of ectopic pregnancy is now commonplace although not yet universal. With increasing sophistication of techniques and fiber optics, many microsurgical procedures can be done through the laparoscope. Recent studies suggest that the fertility rates of laparoscopy and laparotomy are comparable, as are the implications of repeat ectopic pregnancies. Certainly laparoscopy, because of its small incision, results in fewer breakdowns and shorter hospital stays, but the incidence of complications due to retained ectopic tissue is higher.

44. The answer is b. (*Cunningham, 20/e, p 674.*) With velamentous insertion of cord, the umbilical vessels separate in the membranes at a distance from the placental margin, which they reach surrounded only by amnion. It occurs in about 1% of singleton gestations but is quite common in multiple pregnancies. Fetal malformations are more common with velamentous insertion of the umbilical cord. When fetal vessels cross the internal os (vasa previa), rupture of membranes may be accompanied by rupture of a fetal vessel, leading to fetal exsanguination. An increased risk of premature rupture of membranes and of torsion of the umbilical cord has not been described in association with velamentous insertion of cord.

45. The answer is b. (*Mishell, 3/e, pp 452–457.*) Any factor delaying transit of the ovum through the fallopian tube may predispose a patient to ectopic pregnancy. The major predisposing factor in the development of ectopic pregnancies is pelvic inflammatory disease. However, any operative procedure on the fallopian tubes may increase a patient's risk. It appears that tubal sterilizations with laparoscopic fulguration have a higher rate of ectopic pregnancy than tubal ligations performed with clips or rings. Women who have had one ectopic pregnancy are at increased risk of having a second. DES exposure, induction of ovulation, and IUD use increase the possibility of ectopic pregnancies.

46. The answer is d. *(Reece, 2/e, pp 1549, 1700.)* Chorioangiomas are the most common placental tumors, occurring in approximately 1% of placentas. Despite attempts to correlate the presence of these tumors with hydramnios and structural or genetic fetal anomalies, no significant effect on fetal morbidity and mortality has been demonstrated, unless the size of the tumor is very great.

47. The answer is a. *(Rock, 8/e, pp 505–520.)* Although patients with ectopic pregnancies can present with a low-grade febrile response, temperatures above 38°C (100.4°F) are unusual with ectopic pregnancies. Because of placental hormone production from the ectopic pregnancy, the uterus softens and enlarges during the first 3 mo of pregnancy, assays for β-hCG are positive, and nausea can be seen with both ectopic pregnancies and PID. In approximately half of ectopic pregnancies there is an elevated white count up to a maximum of about 30,000. However, leukocytosis is not a sensitive test to separate ectopic pregnancy from pelvic infection.

48. The answer is d. *(Reece, 2/e, pp 1112–1113.)* Hyperemesis gravidarum is intractable vomiting of pregnancy and is associated with disturbed nutrition. Early signs of the disorder include weight loss (up to 5% of body weight) and ketonuria. Because vomiting causes potassium loss, electrocardiographic evidence of potassium depletion, such as inverted T waves and prolonged QT and PR intervals, is usually a later finding. Jaundice also is a later finding and is probably due to fatty infiltration of the liver; occasionally acute hepatic necrosis occurs. Metabolic acidosis is rare. Hypokalemic nephropathy with isosthenuria may occur late. Hypoproteinemia also may result, caused by poor diet as well as by albuminuria. Patients who have hyperemesis gravidarum are best treated (if the disease is early in its course) with parenteral fluids and electrolytes, sedation, rest, vitamins, and antiemetics if necessary. In some cases, isolation of the patient is necessary. Very slow reinstitution of oral feeding is permitted after dehydration and electrolyte disturbances are corrected. Therapeutic abortion may be necessary in rare instances; usually, however, the disease improves spontaneously as pregnancy progresses.

49. The answer is d. *(Gleicher, 3/e, p 163.)* While a 50-rad exposure in the first trimester of pregnancy would be expected to entail a high likelihood of serious fetal damage and wastage, the anticipated fetal exposure for chest x-ray and one film of the lower spine would be less than 1 rad. This is well below the threshold for increased fetal risk, which is generally thought to be 10 rads. High doses of radiation in the first trimester primarily affect developing organ systems such as the heart and limbs; in later pregnancy the brain is more sensitive. The chromosomes are determined at the moment of conception. Radiation does not alter the karyotype, and determination of the karyotype is not normally indicated for a 24-year-old patient. The incidence of leukemia is raised in children receiving radiation therapy or those exposed to the atomic bomb, but not from such a minimal exposure as here.

50. The answer is d. *(Gleicher, 3/e, pp 235–239).* The use of donor eggs has made pregnancy possible in many women in their late 40s, even 50s or more. Although the medical complication risks are higher in older women than in younger women, for a woman in good physical shape, the risks may be acceptable. The principal concern with advancing maternal age has always been the risk of genetic anomalies. By using the eggs of a young donor, these risks can be substantially reduced. Although there is not enough data to say definitively, most experts believe that the age of the egg donor and not the mother is the controlling factor in the risk for aneuploidy in these donor egg cases. With four embryos transferred, yet a quintuplet pregnancy resulting, one of the embryos had to have split into two monozygotic twins. If one is aneuploid, so is the other. Therefore, there are, in fact, approximately four chances that at least one could be aneuploid, and thus the correct answer is approximately 4/550.

51. The answer is e. *(Gleicher, 3/e, pp 239–241.)* Multifetal pregnancy reduction has been shown in numerous individual centers and collaborative studies to substantially reduce morbidity and mortality, particularly among higher-order multiple pregnancies. There is a sharp learning curve in the procedure, and physicians with greater experience have better statistics than those who do not have as much experience. The procedure has been done for up to as many as 12 embryos in a single case, although the data shows very clearly that the higher the starting number, the greater the risk of ultimate loss of the pregnancy and the greater the risk of concomitant prematurity as well. There is complete agreement in the literature that with quadruplets or more as a starting number, reduction to twins vastly improves outcome for the remaining fetuses. There is controversy, but most people believe that the same is also true for triplets. α fetoprotein measurements are not usable following reduction, as the levels will always be high secondary to the demised fetuses.

52. The answer is b. *(Gleicher, 3/e, pp 203–204.)* It has been shown in numerous studies that nuchal translucency measured between 10 and 13 wk is a useful marker for increased risk of chromosome abnormalities such as, but not limited to, Down syndrome. The larger the nuchal translucency, the greater risk of other adverse pregnancy outcomes, including fetal demise, cardiac abnormalities, and other genetic syndromes, even if the karyotype is normal. The nuchal translucency will almost always disappear by 15 wk; this does not reduce the risk of there being an aneuploid condition, although cystic hygromas in the second trimester are primarily associated with Turner syndrome. In the first trimester, nuchal translucencies most likely indicate Down syndrome, followed by trisomy 18 and then Turner syndrome.

GENETICS, FETAL INFECTIONS, CONGENITAL ANOMALIES, PRENATAL DIAGNOSIS, AND ULTRASOUND

Questions

DIRECTIONS: Each group of questions below consists of lettered options followed by numbered items. For each numbered item, select the appropriate lettered option(s). Each lettered option may be used once, more than once, or not at all. **Choose exactly the number of options indicated following each item.**

Items 53–60

For each situation below, select the appropriate inheritance pattern.

a. Autosomal dominant
b. Autosomal recessive
c. X-linked recessive
d. Codominant
e. Multifactorial

53. Glucose-6-phosphate dehydrogenase (G6PD) deficiency (**SELECT 1 PATTERN**)

54. Neurofibromatosis (**SELECT 1 PATTERN**)

55. Becker muscular dystrophy (**SELECT 1 PATTERN**)

56. Haplotypes (**SELECT 1 PATTERN**)

57. 21-hydroxylase deficiency congenital adrenal hypoplasia (**SELECT 1 PATTERN**)

58. Ornithine transcarbamylase deficiency (**SELECT 1 PATTERN**)

59. Cystic fibrosis (**SELECT 1 PATTERN**)

60. Huntington's disease (**SELECT 1 PATTERN**)

DIRECTIONS: Each item below contains a question or incomplete statement followed by suggested responses. Select the **one best** response to each question.

61. A woman and her husband are both carriers for Tay-Sachs disease. The woman is pregnant with dizygotic twins. The chance that at least one of the twins will be affected with Tay-Sachs disease is

a. 25%
b. 44%
c. 50%
d. 56%
e. 75%

62. Achondroplasia is characterized by which of the following statements?

a. The inheritance pattern is autosomal recessive
b. New mutations account for 50% of all cases
c. Cesarean section is rarely necessary
d. Affected women rarely live to reproductive age
e. Spinal deformaties lead to cord compression

63. Which of the following statements regarding cystic fibrosis is true?

a. The ΔF508 gene is more common in Jewish than Scottish patients
b. If ΔF508 is not present, this eliminates carrier risk
c. ΔF508 can be used to diagnose 70% of fetuses at risk
d. With multiple markers, a fetus who has one positive and one negative chromosome 7 has a 1/900 risk of cystic fibrosis
e. If ΔF508 is present on one chromosome 7, the fetus must be a carrier of cystic fibrosis

64. The third-trimester fetus of a mother with a balanced 13/13 translocation would have what likelihood of having an abnormal chromosome karyotype?

a. 2%
b. 10%
c. 25%
d. 50%
e. 100%

65. The ultrasound image below is representative of

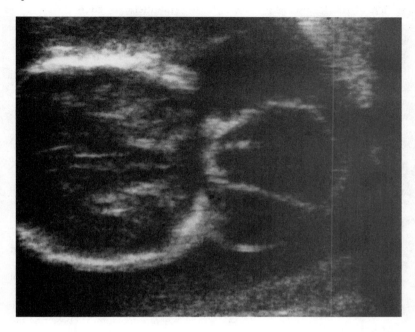

a. A cystic hygroma
b. An encephalocele
c. Hydrocephalus
d. Anencephaly
e. None of the above

66. A 24-year-old white woman has a maternal serum α fetoprotein (MSAFP) at 17 wk gestation of 6.0 multiples of the median (MOM). The next step should be

a. A second MSAFP test
b. Ultrasound examination
c. Amniocentesis
d. Amniography
e. Recommendation of termination

67. A 32-year-old has a fetus at increased risk for Down syndrome. Which of the following is considered only after the MOM is calculated for Down syndrome risks?

a.   Maternal weight
b.   Race
c.   Maternal age
d.   Gestational age
e.   Multiple gestations

68. Advantages of ultrasound nuchal translucency over biochemical screening for Down syndrome include

a.   Uses transvaginal approach
b.   More consistent measurements than lab tests
c.   Better in multiple gestation
d.   Wide gestational age range
e.   More convenient for patients

69. A 41-year-old had a baby with Down syndrome 10 years ago. She is anxious to know the chromosome status of her fetus in a current pregnancy. The test she can have that has the fastest lab processing time for karyotype is

a.   Amniocentesis
b.   Cordocentesis
c.   Chorionic villus sampling (CVS)
d.   Doppler flow ultrasound
e.   Cystic hygroma aspiration

70. A baby is born with ambiguous genitalia. Which of the following statements is true?

a.   A karyotype is rarely needed
b.   Evaluation should be done by 1 mo of age
c.   It is sometimes associated with a history of a previous sibling with congenital adrenal hyperplasia (CAH)
d.   A thorough physical examination can usually decide the true sex
e.   Laparotomy or laparoscopy is required for CAH cases

71. A 39-year-old wants first-trimester prenatal diagnosis. Advantages of early amniocentesis over CVS include

a.   Amniocentesis can be performed earlier in pregnancy
b.   Amniocentesis is usually less painful
c.   Second-trimester diagnosis allows for safer termination of pregnancy when termination is chosen by the patient
d.   CVS has a lower complication rate than midtrimester amniocentesis
e.   CVS has a lower complication rate than first trimester amniocentesis

Items 72–78

Match the descriptions with the appropriate marker.

a. MSAFP
b. Beta subunit of human chorionic gonadotropin (β-hCG)
c. Estriol
d. Pregnancy-associated placental proteins-A (PAPP-A)
e. Urea-resistant nuclear alkaline phosphatase (URNAP)
f. Nicked β-hCG
g. β-hCG degradation protein

72. Elevated in Down syndrome and currently used (**SELECT 1 MARKER**)

73. Labile proteins with high sensitivity (**SELECT 1 MARKER**)

74. Better in first trimester than second (**SELECT 1 MARKER**)

75. Detector of neural tube defect (**SELECT 1 MARKER**)

76. Urine test (**SELECT 1 MARKER**)

77. Highest sensitivity for Down syndrome, but labor intensive (**SELECT 1 MARKER**)

78. Least useful of triple-screen parameters (**SELECT 1 MARKER**)

Items 79–87

For each ultrasonogram, **SELECT 1 DIAGNOSIS OR DIAGNOSTIC INDICATOR.**

a. Obstructed urethra and bladder
b. Nonspinal marker for spina bifida
c. Indication of highest likelihood of a chromosomal abnormality
d. Marker for Down syndrome (trisomy 21)
e. Common marker for trisomies 18 and 21
f. Osteogenesis imperfecta
g. Mesomelic dwarfism
h. Anencephaly
i. Prune belly syndrome
j. Hydrocephalus
k. Spina bifida with meningocele

79.

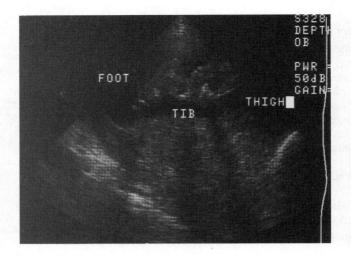

80.

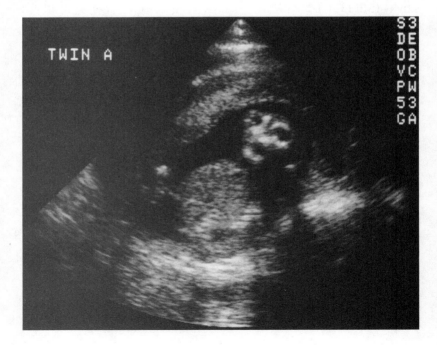

81.

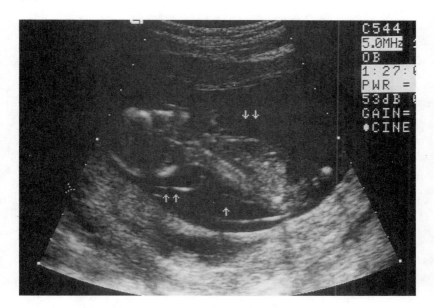

82.

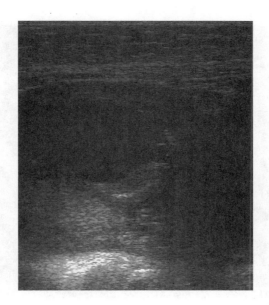

83.

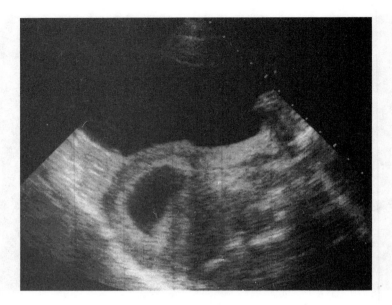

84.

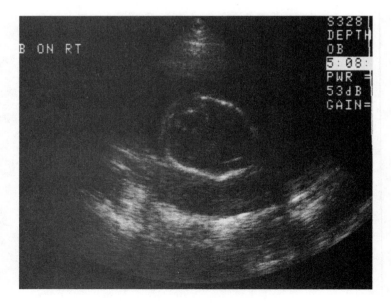

85.

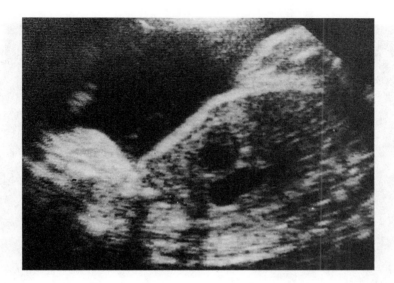

86.

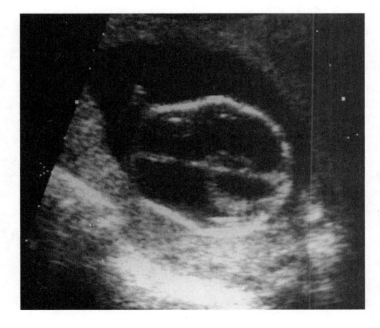

87.

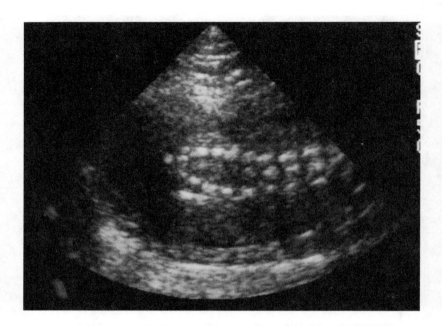

Items 88–94

Match each description with the correct technique.

a. Transabdominal CVS
b. Transcervical CVS
c. Early amniocentesis
d. Traditional amniocentesis
e. Cordocentesis

88. Contraindicated with herpes infection **(SELECT 1 TECHNIQUE)**

89. Useful for measuring fetal immunoglobulin M (IgM) levels **(SELECT 1 TECHNIQUE)**

90. Useful for diagnosing fetal anemias **(SELECT 1 TECHNIQUE)**

91. Clinical experience of less than 10,000 cases **(SELECT 1 TECHNIQUE)**

92. Ability to detect neural tube defects **(SELECT 1 TECHNIQUE)**

93. Culture failure rate of approximately 5% **(SELECT 1 TECHNIQUE)**

94. Membrane tenting is a complication **(SELECT 1 TECHNIQUE)**

95. True statements about a pregnant woman who has phenylketonuria (PKU) include which of the following?

a. If the father carries the gene, the risk that the child will be affected is 25%
b. Phenylketonuria can be detected prenatally by measuring phenylalanine (Phe) levels in chorionic villi
c. Persons with phenylketonuria rarely survive to the reproductive years
d. Genetically normal children born to mothers who have phenylketonuria are frequently mentally retarded
e. PKU-induced mental retardation can be prevented by diet starting by 1 year of age

96. The most frequent pathogen currently implicated in infectious causes of early abortion is

a. *Brucella abortus*
b. *Listeria monocytogenes*
c. *Toxoplasma gondii*
d. *Mycoplasma hominis*
e. *Streptococcus agalacture*

97. The initial maternal immunologic response to a primary rubella infection is the elaboration of

a. Immunoglobulin A
b. Immunoglobulin D
c. Immunoglobulin M
d. Immunoglobulin G
e. Complement-fixation antibodies

98. A 33-year-old has an infection in pregnancy. Which of the following is a reinfection, and therefore not a risk to the fetus?

a. Group B coxsackievirus
b. Rubella virus
c. Chickenpox virus
d. Shingles
e. Herpesvirus hominis type 2

99. Viremia and the presence of rubella virus in the throat of infected persons bear which of the following relationships to the onset of the rubella rash?

a. They precede the rash by 5 to 7 days
b. They precede the rash by 1 to 2 days
c. They occur coincidentally with the rash
d. They occur 1 to 2 days after the rash
e. They bear no consistent relationship to the onset of the rash

100. A pregnant woman is discovered to be an asymptomatic carrier of *Neisseria gonorrhoeae*. A year ago, she was treated with penicillin for a gonococcal infection and developed a severe allergic reaction. Treatment of choice at this time would be

a. Tetracycline
b. Ampicillin
c. Spectinomycin
d. Chloramphenicol
e. Penicillin

101. Vaccines are contraindicated in pregnancy, even following maternal exposure, for which of the following diseases?

a. Rabies
b. Tetanus
c. Typhoid
d. Hepatitis B
e. Measles

102. True statements concerning vaccines include

a. Inactivated vaccines are hazardous to the mother
b. Cases of congenital rubella syndrome have been reported in fetuses born to mothers who were immunized early in pregnancy
c. Inactivated vaccines are hazardous to the fetus
d. The polio virus has the ability to spread from the vaccine to susceptible persons in the immediate environment
e. Nonimmune pregnant women who are exposed to children who recently received the measles-mumps-rubella (MMR) vaccine are at high risk of delivery of an infected fetus

103. A 22-year-old has just had a baby diagnosed with toxoplasmosis. You try to determine what her risk factors were. The highest risk associations would be

a. Eating raw meat
b. Eating raw fish
c. Having a dog
d. Being English
e. Having viral infections in early pregnancy

104. Appropriate tests following an elevated maternal toxoplasmosis titer include

a. Maternal total IgM titers
b. Amniotic fluid toxoplasmosis-specific immunoglobulin G (IgG) titers
c. Amniotic fluid toxoplasmosis-specific IgM titers
d. Fetal blood toxoplasmosis-specific IgG titers by cordocentesis
e. Fetal blood toxoplasmosis-specific IgM titers by cordocentesis

Items 105–108

Select the antibiotic most frequently associated with the following fetal side effects.

a. Tetracycline
b. Streptomycin
c. Nitrofurantoin
d. Chloramphenicol
e. Sulfonamides

105. Hypoplasia and staining of fetal teeth **(SELECT 1 ANTIBIOTIC)**

106. Kernicterus of the newborn **(SELECT 1 ANTIBIOTIC)**

107. Fetal high-tone hearing loss **(SELECT 1 ANTIBIOTIC)**

108. Gray baby syndrome **(SELECT 1 ANTIBIOTIC)**

Items 109–113

For each description that follows, select the microorganism with which it is most likely to be associated.

a. Rubella virus
b. Cytomegalovirus
c. Group A β-hemolytic streptococci
d. Group B β-hemolytic streptococci
e. *Toxoplasma gondii*

109. This organism may cause epidemics of puerperal sepsis **(SELECT 1 MICROORGANISM)**

110. A pregnant woman may become infected with this organism by contact with infected cat feces **(SELECT 1 MICROORGANISM)**

111. An effective vaccine exists for the prevention of adult infection with this organism **(SELECT 1 MICROORGANISM)**

112. This organism is an important cause of neonatal sepsis and meningitis **(SELECT 1 MICROORGANISM)**

113. Vaccination should be administered postpartum to nonimmune women **(SELECT 1 MICROORGANISM)**

Items 114–118

The safety of immunization during pregnancy is a matter of concern and controversy that has prompted the American College of Obstetricians and Gynecologists to offer specific recommendations for the use of immunization therapy for pregnant women. For each disease, select the recommendation regarding vaccination with which it is most likely to be associated.

a. Recommended if the underlying disease is serious
b. Recommended after exposure or before travel to endemic areas
c. Not routinely recommended, but mandatory during an epidemic
d. Contraindicated unless exposure to the disease is unavoidable
e. Contraindicated

114. Poliomyelitis **(SELECT 1 RECOMMENDATION)**

115. Mumps **(SELECT 1 RECOMMENDATION)**

116. Influenza **(SELECT 1 RECOMMENDATION)** .

117. Rubella **(SELECT 1 RECOMMENDATION)**

118. Hepatitis A **(SELECT 1 RECOMMENDATION)**

Items 119–122

For each of the syndromes or diseases below, choose the virus responsible when the fetus is exposed in utero.

a. Cytomegalovirus
b. Rubella
c. Varicella zoster
d. Rubeola
e. Hepatitis B

119. Cataracts, cardiac defects, deafness **(SELECT 1 VIRUS)**

120. Cirrhosis, primary hepatocellular carcinoma **(SELECT 1 VIRUS)**

121. Cicatricial skin lesions, limb hypoplasia, rudimentary digits **(SELECT 1 VIRUS)**

122. Microcephaly, intracerebral calcifications, hepatosplenomegaly **(SELECT 1 VIRUS)**

Items 123–124

Certain diseases in pregnant women are associated with fetal congenital anomalies. Match each description with the correct diseases.

a. Rubella
b. Mumps
c. Acquired immune deficiency syndrome (AIDS)
d. Cytomegalovirus
e. Influenza

123. Associated with fetal congenital anomalies (**SELECT 2 DISEASES**)

124. Not associated with fetal congenital anomalies (**SELECT 3 DISEASES**)

125. A syndrome of multiple congenital anomalies including microcephaly, cardiac anomalies, and growth retardation has been described in children of women who are heavy users of

a. Amphetamines
b. Barbiturates
c. Heroin
d. Methadone
e. Ethyl alcohol

126. Congenital heart malformations occur with exposure to teratogenic agents at what postmenstrual age?

a. 2 to 3 wk
b. 4 to 5 wk
c. 6 to 8 wk
d. 9 to 12 wk
e. 13 to 15 wk

Items 127–128

Match each description with the correct drug.

a. Erythromycin
b. Tetracycline
c. Penicillin
d. Chloramphenicol
e. Ampicillin
f. Trimethoprim-sulfamethoxazole (Bactrim)

127. Safe in all trimesters (**SELECT 3 DRUGS**)

128. Unsafe in all trimesters (**SELECT 2 DRUGS**)

129. Prenatal treatment of birth defects will not ameliorate the clinical situation for which of the following?

a. Obstructed bladder outflow
b. Porencephalic cysts
c. Cardiac arrhythmias
d. Adrenogenital syndrome
e. Diaphragmatic hernia

Items 130–132

For all of the following, match the correct concept to the clinical data below

a. Sensitivity
b. Specificity
c. Positive predictive value
d. Negative predictive value

130. An epidemiologist is studying the usefulness of a new test for human immunodeficiency virus (HIV) and wants to know what percentage of patients who have AIDS will test positive for it with the new procedure

131. A patient wishes to know, given her negative pap smear, what is the likelihood that she will, in fact, not have cervical cancer

132. A patient has a positive screen for Down syndrome and wants to know what is the chance that the fetus is, in fact, affected

Items 133–135

For all of the following, match the correct concept to the clinical data below

a. Diagnostic test
b. Screening test

133. A 42-year-old woman undergoes biochemical screening that reveals a Down syndrome risk of 1 in 4

134. A 27-year-old woman undergoes an ultrasound at 10 wk gestation that reveals a nuchal translucency of 4 mm

135. A 26-year-old woman undergoes an ultrasound at 18 wk gestation that reveals a lumbar-sacral meningomyelocele

GENETICS, FETAL INFECTIONS, CONGENITAL ANOMALIES, PRENATAL DIAGNOSIS, AND ULTRASOUND

Answers

53–60. The answers are 53-c, 54-a, 55-c, 56-d, 57-b, 58-c, 59-b, 60-a. *(Korf, pp 5, 132–161.)* Glucose-6-phosphate dehydrogenase (G6PD) deficiency is X-linked recessive and is found predominantly in males of African and Mediterranean origin. Although the causes of clinical manifestations in G6PD deficiency are multifactorial (e.g., sulfa drugs), the inheritance is not. Neurofibromatosis, whose occurrence is often sporadic (i.e., a spontaneous mutation in 50%), is inherited as an autosomal dominant trait once the gene is in a family. The severity of the condition can be quite variable even within the same family. Becker muscular dystrophy, an X-linked recessive disorder, is allelic to Duchenne muscular dystrophy, but has much milder manifestations. The human leukocyte antigens (HLAs) (four from each parent) are all expressed and therefore do not show any dominance in their expression. Certain combinations of haplotypes are associated with some disease conditions (such as 21-hydroxylase deficiency congenital adrenal hyperplasia, which is autosomal recessive) in that they occur much more commonly than would be expected by chance; however, such associations do not, alone, define inheritance. Ornithine transcarbamylase deficiency is an X-linked trait observed mostly in heterozygotic females because the hemizygous males do not survive. The females are protein intolerant and sometimes have diminished intelligence. Cystic fibrosis is the most common autosomal recessive disorder in the white European population, and Huntington's disease is autosomal dominant.

61. The answer is b. *(Korf, pp 36–38, 319.)* Tay-Sachs disease is an autosomal recessive disease. In any single conception, the chance that a fetus is affected is one-half that the gene is donated by the mother times one-half that the gene is donated by the father, or 25%. If there are two successive pregnancies, or fraternal twins in one pregnancy, the chances are independent probabilities whose risks are multiplied. To analyze the question of whether at least one fetus is affected—which is usually the true clinical concern—the easiest approach is to look at the probability that neither will be affected and then subtract that from 1. In other words, the chance that there will be an unaffected fetus in the first pregnancy is three-quarters (one-quarter unaffected, two-quarters carrier). The chance that there will be an unaffected fetus in both pregnancies is therefore three-quarters times three-quarters, or 56%. Therefore, the chance that there will be at least one affected pregnancy is 1 minus the risk of no pregnancies, or 44%. Had the twin pregnancy been monozygotic, either both twins or neither twin would be affected, and the risk would be 25% for an affected pregnancy.

62. The answer is e. *(Jones, 5/e, pp 346–351.)* Achondroplasia, a congenital disorder of cartilage formation characterized by dwarfism, is associated with an autosomal dominant pattern of inheritance. However, mutations account for 90% of all cases of the disorder. Affected women almost always require cesarean section because of the distorted shape of their pelves. Achondroplastic fetuses, when prenatally diagnosed, should also be delivered by cesarean section to minimize trauma to the fetal neck. Women who have achondroplasia and receive adequate treatment for its associated complications, including the neurologic signs of cord compression due to spinal deformity, generally have a normal life expectancy.

63. The answer is d. *(Remoin, 3/e, pp 2685–2717.)* Cystic fibrosis is the most common autosomal recessive disease seen in the white population and is particularly prevalent among people of northern European ancestry. In 1986 it was discovered that the cystic fibrosis gene was on chromosome 7, and in 1989 the exact location of the cystic fibrosis gene—called the cystic fibrosis transmembrane conductance regulator—was delineated. Analysis shows that approximately 70% of cystic fibrosis is related to a deficiency of the protein associated with a deletion at residue 508 of the mature protein. Such a deletion is now diagnosable by oligonucleotype probes and is called ΔF508. ΔF508 is seen in varying degrees in carriers of cystic fibrosis. For patients with cystic fibrosis who are black, Jewish, or of Spanish origin, for example, the proportion of cases associated with

ΔF508 is considerably lower than for those having Scottish, Irish, or German ancestries. If a patient does not have the ΔF508 deletion, carrier status can never be eliminated because the patient still may have another deletion or DNA change that causes cystic fibrosis. While an average 70% of individual chromosomes that are carrier chromosomes for cystic fibrosis have the ΔF508 deletion, oligonucleotype probes will not pick up 70% of the cases. The chance that a low-risk patient has inherited cystic fibrosis genes from both chromosomes in meiosis is 70% that the inheritance comes from the father times 70% that the inheritance also comes from the mother; in other words, only approximately 49% of low-risk cases will be detected. However, if the ΔF508 deletion is present on both chromosome 7s, the fetus does have cystic fibrosis. If the ΔF508 deletion is present on only one chromosome 7, there is still a risk that the non-ΔF508 chromosome may in fact carry cystic fibrosis. Family pedigree and history may be helpful, e.g., if there is another affected person with the same chromosome complement; however, there may also be considerable clinical uncertainty. There are now over 600 known mutations causing cystic fibrosis. With multiple markers now available, the percentage of detection with 32 markers approaches 90%, but there is still great controversy as to when universal screening of low-risk pregnancies will be appropriate. However, a fetus that is negative/negative is at only a 1/200,000 risk, while a fetus that is positive/negative is at 1/900.

64. The answer is e. (*Korf, pp 143–144, 187–189.*) Carriers of balanced translocations of the same chromosome are phenotypically normal. However, in the process of gamete formation (either sperm or ova), the translocated chromosome cannot divide and therefore the meiosis products end up with either two copies or no copies of the particular chromosome. In the former case, fertilization leads to trisomy of that chromosome. Many trisomies are lethal in utero. Trisomies of 13, 18, and 21 lead to classic syndromes. In the latter case, a monosomy is produced, and all except for monosomy X (Turner syndrome) are lethal in utero.

65. The answer is b. (*Fleisher, 5/e, pp 216–223. Timor-Tritsch, p 325.*) An encephalocele is an outpouching of neural tissue through a defect in the skull. A cystic hygroma, with which encephalocele can often be confused on ultrasound, emerges from the base of the neck with an intact skull present. Hydrocephalus is related to the size of the lateral ventricles. Anencephaly would require absence of a much larger proportion of the skull with diminished neural tissues.

66. The answer is b. *(Gleicher, 3/e, pp 199–205.)* The recommended sequence for an MSAFP screening program for 1000 hypothetical patients would normally produce about 30 with an elevated level (2.5 MOM) on the first MSAFP. If the patient does not have an extremely elevated value (i.e., the value is <4.0 MOM) and is relatively early in pregnancy (<19 wk gestation), a second MSAFP value is usually drawn. About two-thirds of these patients will have an elevated test or will be very high the first time. Those that are normal a second time drop back into the normal population. However, if the value is extremely high (≥4.0 MOM) or if the gestational age is approaching the limit of options for termination of pregnancy (19+ wk), most programs then skip a second test and go directly on to ultrasound and possibly amniocentesis. A thorough ultrasound on patients with two elevations or one very high elevation will reveal an obvious reason for the elevation in about 10 of 30 patients. These reasons may include anencephaly, twins, wrong gestational age of the fetus, or a fetal demise. The approximately 20 patients with no obvious cause for their elevations should then be offered counseling and amniocentesis. There is debate in the literature that, if the ultrasound is normal, amniocentesis is unnecessary. We believe that is appropriate to adjust odds, but that ultrasound can never be perfect. Of patients without a benign explanation, about 5% have an elevated amniotic fluid α fetoprotein (AFP) and positive acetylcholinesterase. Such patients will have a greater than 99% chance of having a baby with an open neural tube defect or other serious malformations, such as a ventral wall defect. Amniography is an outmoded procedure in which radiopaque dye is injected into the amniotic cavity for the purpose of taking x-rays. Under no circumstances whatsoever should termination of pregnancy be recommended on the basis of MSAFP testing alone. MSAFP is only a screening test used to define who is at risk and requires further testing; it is never diagnostic per se.

67. The answer is c. *(Gleicher, 3/e, pp 199–205.)* The association of low MSAFP values and increased risk of chromosomal abnormalities, most notably Down syndrome, has been known since the mid-1980s. All the listed factors are important in MSAFP screening. However, maternal age is not used as a criterion in determining the multiple of the median (MOM), but is used once the MOM has been determined. Because AFP is a fetal product, if it is distributed over a larger mother, the effective serum concentration is lower. Therefore a maternal weight correction is used to adjust for differing plasma volumes. The race of the patient is important because, for reasons that are unclear, black patients have slightly higher levels of MSAFP than do white patients despite the fact that the risk of neural tube defects in the black population is lower than that of white patients. A separate database for black and white patients is the most optimal way of handling such data. Gestational age is important because AFP values normally rise in maternal serum with advancing gestational age. A significant discrepancy between a patient's opinion of gestational age and actual gestational age may explain a seemingly abnormal result. Multiple gestations are important because if there are two or more fetuses, the value of AFP seen normally will be higher. In most programs an upper cutoff point of 4.5 MOM is used for known twins, and a lower cutoff point of 1.0 MOM is common for increased risk of chromosomal abnormalities.

68. The answer is c. *(Gleicher, 3/e, pp 203–205.)* The ultrasound nuchal translucency (NT) is now appreciated as a sensitive marker for Down syndrome and other aneuploidies between 10 and 13 wk. Outside that range, the NT disappears. Although some centers have had superb results, others have not done well. Blood free β-hCG and PAPP-A in the first trimester, and double (AFP and hCG) or triple (AFP, hCG, and estriol at 15 to 20 wk) are statistically comparable. The combination of NT and first-trimester biochemistry will likely be the optimal approach. Biochemistry does not work well for multiple gestations. Ultrasound can also detect structural anomalies, but often high-quality ultrasound services require patients to travel long distances, whereas blood can be shipped from essentially anywhere to a competent lab.

69. The answer is c. *(Gleicher, 3/e, pp 178–190.)* Amniocentesis, cordocentesis, cystic hygroma aspiration, and chorionic villus sampling are techniques of obtaining fetal tissues that are amenable to cytogenetic analysis. Amniotic fluid cells require tissue culture to obtain adequate cell numbers for analysis. Chorionic villi can be harvested directly for extremely rapid diagnosis or can be cultured for higher banding (increased detail). Fetal blood obtained by cordocentesis or percutaneous umbilical blood sampling (PUBS) requires 2 to 3 days of culturing before a karyotype is obtained. Doppler flow ultrasound is used to assess blood flow through fetal vessels, but is not a substitute for direct analysis of tissue.

70. The answer is c. *(Gidwani, pp 89–96.)* Ambiguous genitalia at birth are a medical emergency, not only for psychological reasons for the parents but also because hirsute female infants with congenital adrenal hyperplasia (CAH) may die if undiagnosed. CAH is an autosomally inherited disease of adrenal failure that causes hyponatremia and hyperkalemia because of lack of mineralocorticoids. Although a thorough physical examination is helpful, especially for inguinal testes, other tests that are required include a karyotype, serum electrolytes, and blood or urine assays for progesterone, 17α-hydroxyprogesterone, and androgens such as dehydroepiandrosterone sulfate. Radiologic studies are usually not needed, but a laparotomy is sometimes necessary for ectopic gonadectomy.

71. The answer is e. *(Gleicher, 3/e, pp 178–190.)* Chorionic villus sampling (CVS) has many theoretical and practical advantages over amniocentesis, including its earlier performance and quicker results. CVS is performed as a transcervical catheter procedure the majority of the time; therefore, there are no needles and the procedure is painless. Suction terminations during the first trimester are safer than prostaglandin and other second-trimester techniques. However, CVS does have a somewhat higher complication rate. In the most experienced hands, midtrimester genetic amniocentesis probably carries about a 1/300 risk and CVS probably has a 1/150 to 1/200 risk. Early or first-trimester amniocentesis has a complication rate higher than that for CVS, and has been shown to have an increased risk of talipes.

72–78. The answers are 72-b, 73-f, 74-d, 75-a, 76-g, 77-e, 78-c. *(Gleicher, 3/e, pp 199–205.)* The uses of multiple markers for biochemical screening for fetuses who carry chromosomal abnormalities such as Down syndrome or neural tube defects have become more sophisticated in the past several years. Since MSAFP screening was introduced nearly 30 years ago for neural tube defects, it has remained the only biochemical marker for such anomalies. Low MSAFP was introduced in the mid-1980s for chromosomal abnormalities, although it is now known that elevated β-hCG is a much better marker for Down syndrome than MSAFP or the third analyte in the triple-screen paradigm, estriol. There is considerable debate about the utility of estriol, i.e., whether the two markers MSAFP and hCG are as good as or better than also adding the third marker estriol. PAPP-A, a newer marker, has been shown to be very effective in the first trimester, but useless in the second trimester. The single best test may turn out to be URNAP, but currently the test is not automated and therefore not useful as a mass screening tool. Nicked β-hCG is a structurally abnormal form of β-hCG that has high sensitivity but is very labile. Urinary β degradation core is promising as a new marker.

79–87. The answers are 79-f, 80-h, 81-e, 82-a, 83-c, 84-b, 85-d, 86-j, 87-k. *(Benacerraf, pp 229–235. Fleisher, 5/e, pp 471–472.)* The diagnosis of osteogenesis imperfecta can be made by visualizing fractures in utero by ultrasound. The ultrasound in question 79 shows a crumpling of the tibia and fibula and curvature of the thigh such that proper extension of the foot does not occur. A molecular diagnosis of osteogenesis imperfecta can be made on a case-by-case family basis by looking for particular deletions in the molecular structure of collagen. It is not uncommon for patients with osteogenesis imperfecta type II—the lethal form—to have dozens of fractures before birth. Osteogenesis imperfecta types I and III, which are compatible with life and often cause blue sclerae (type I), are often not detectable before birth.

The ultrasonogram in question 80 was done at approximately 15 wk gestation and shows two orbits, a mouth, and a central nose, but there is clearly no forehead and no cranial contents. Even a relatively inexperienced sonographer using average equipment available in the early 1990s would be able to pick up anencephaly. Anencephaly is, of course, incompatible with life and is the only condition for which a termination of pregnancy is generally permissible at any gestational age.

The ultrasonogram in question 81 shows a 13-wk-old fetus with a large nuchal translucency (double arrows) and beginning hydrops, sometimes called a cystic hygroma. Increasing experience with early ultrasonograms has demonstrated that cystic hygromas occur in 1% to 2% of patients. In the second and third trimesters, cystic hygromas are commonly associated with Turner syndrome (45,X). The earlier in pregnancy they are seen, however, the more likely the diagnosis is related to trisomy 21, trisomy 18, or trisomy 13, which are collectively found on karyotype in approximately 50% of the cases. Of those cases that are chromosomally normal, most of these nuchal translucencies disappear and the fetus goes on to have perfectly normal development.

In question 82, the transverse cut through the bladder shows mega-cystis (i.e., the bladder is markedly enlarged) and the distal portion of the urethra can be visualized up to the point of urinary blockage. The blocked urethra acts as a dam that causes the bladder to fill up, then the ureters, and finally the kidneys (hydronephrosis). There is oligohydramnios noted in this picture because by 16 wk—the gestational age at which this picture was taken—the vast majority of amniotic fluid comes from fetal urine. Left untreated, these babies will often develop prune belly syndrome and show kidney and abdominal wall damage. The cause of death, however, is pulmonary because the oligohydramnios does not allow for proper lung development. When these babies are born, they die from pulmonary causes; they do not live long enough to die from renal causes.

The ultrasonogram in question 83 was performed at approximately 8 wk after the last menstrual period and shows a placenta but no fetal pole—the classic blighted ovum. Traditionally 50% of first-trimester spontaneous abortions are said to be chromosomally abnormal. However, more recent evidence suggests that, particularly with advancing age of the mother (i.e., in women who are likely to have early ultrasonography for potential CVS), the risk of fetal chromosomal abnormalities is in fact much higher, in many cases approaching even 90% of first-trimester spontaneous abortions. A CVS catheter can be seen entering the placenta at the top of the uterus to obtain a postmortem CVS. Recent experience has also shown that the highest likelihood of obtaining a karyotype on a fetal demise is by obtaining tissue by CVS at the time of diagnosis rather than waiting to culture abortus material after the uterine contents have been evacuated.

The cross section through the fetal head in question 84 shows a classic lemon sign; that is, there is a frontal bosselation of the forehead such that the sides of the forehead are actually pulled in. This is because of the pull on the cisterna magna from spina bifida that is distorting the intracranial contents. This so-called lemon sign has a very high degree of sensitivity, although it is not perfect. Furthermore, the lemon sign disappears in the third trimester and is therefore not useful late in pregnancy.

The longitudinal ultrasonogram in question 85 shows the double bubble related to duodenal atresia. The two bubbles are the stomach and the jejunum. This finding is classic for trisomy 21. Approximately one-third of fetuses who have this finding will in fact be found to have trisomy 21. This risk, of course, is very high and is an automatic indication for offering prenatal diagnosis by either amniocentesis, CVS, or cordocentesis to document the chromosomes regardless of any other indication the patient may have.

88–94. The answers are 88-b, 89-e, 90-e, 91-c, 92-d, 93-c, 94-c. *(Gleicher, 3/e, pp 178–190.)* Chorionic villus sampling has become a routine part of prenatal diagnosis and is offered at centers around the world. Two different approaches are used: transcervical and transabdominal. The advantages of the transcervical approach include less patient discomfort and larger sample size. Transabdominal CVS is preferable for late gestational ages and in patients with vaginal or cervical infections. The question of an increased risk of limb reduction defects in patients having CVS was raised in the early 1990s, but convincing data now shows that there is no increased risk for any birth defects whatsoever for CVS patients versus the general population when CVS is performed at the usual gestational ages, i.e., after 9 wk. There may be a slightly increased risk for experimental cases performed at 6 to 7 wk gestation, but this is not a routine time to perform the procedure. Fetal blood sampling by cordocentesis permits the diagnosis of fetal infection and aneuploidy by analysis of blood constituents.

Early amniocentesis has been proposed as an alternative to chorionic villus sampling (CVS). The first major problem with this is that there has been no uniform definition of exactly what an early amniocentesis is. The author has adopted the terminology of *routine amniocentesis* for 14 wk gestation or more, *early amniocentesis* for weeks 12 and 13, and *very early amniocentesis* for less than 12 wk. It is well known that the overall loss rate for any procedure is primarily a function of the gestational age at which it is performed, which reflects natural losses and has nothing to do with the procedure. Thus there must be extreme caution in interpreting any data. CVS has been performed in over 300,000 cases and has a documented procedure loss rate of between 0.5% and 1%. Early and very early amniocenteses have only been performed in a few thousand cases, most of which are clustered at the higher end of the gestational age curve. It is thus very difficult to assess the true risks of procedures at comparable ages. Also, there appears to be an increased role of talipes (club foot) in early amniocenteses done before 13 wk. It is also known that there are many fewer cells in early amniotic fluid than there are later, which makes the time of culture growth longer and the growth culture failure rate of 5% much higher than that seen for regular amniocentesis or CVS procedures. Molecular and biochemical analyses require many cells, and even the smallest solid tissue specimen has many more cells than large volumes of amniotic fluid, which makes chorionic villi preferable for such analyses. Neural tube defects can be diagnosed by α fetoprotein and acetylcholinesterase, which can be measured in amniotic fluid but not in chorionic villi. Obtaining an early amniocentesis specimen can be complicated by tenting of the membranes, as the amnion and chorion are poorly fused prior to 13 to 14 wk.

95. The answer is d. *(Jones, 5/e, pp 580–581, 686.)* If a woman who has phenylketonuria (PKU), an autosomal recessive disorder, marries a carrier for this disease, the chance that offspring will be affected is 50%. Phenylketonuria can now be detected prenatally through the use of DNA/molecular techniques. Screening of newborns and early institution of low-phenylalanine diets (<3 wk) have made it possible for affected persons to reach adulthood. It has become apparent that a high frequency of mental retardation exists in children of mothers who have phenylketonuria, even if these children do not themselves have the disease. Retardation in these children presumably is related to intrauterine exposure to high phenylalanine levels in the maternal blood. Whether or not a mother with PKU can be compelled to follow a diet for the sake of the developing fetus will be a significant ethical debate.

96. The answer is d. *(Speroff, 6/e, pp 519. Gleicher, 3/e, 741–742.)* There have been increased numbers of investigations linking mycoplasma infections with early abortions. There may be a role for preconceptual tetracycline therapy in couples with histories of habitual abortions. However, tetracycline agents are not generally considered appropriate in pregnancy.

97. The answer is c. *(Gleicher, 3/e, pp 568–557.)* The first response to a primary infection of rubella and other viruses is the elaboration of immunoglobulin M (IgM). Although IgM, once produced, is present for at least several weeks, rising levels of immunoglobulin G (IgG) account for the fact that IgG eventually constitutes nearly all antibody detected in the serum. Complement-fixation antibodies usually appear 7 to 10 days after appearance of the rubella rash.

98. The answer is d. *(Rodeck, p 858.)* A mild group B coxsackievirus infection of the mother during the antepartum period may give rise to a virulent infection in the newborn, sometimes resulting in a fatal encephalomyocarditis. A maternal rubella infection may cause neonatal hepatosplenomegaly, petechial rash, and jaundice; in addition, viral shedding may last for months or years. Herpes zoster, the causative agent of varicella (chickenpox), is an especially dangerous organism for the newborn. Varicella is rare in pregnancy, but if it occurs shortly before delivery, the viremia may spread to the fetus before protective maternal antibodies have had a chance to form. Congenital varicella can be fatal to the newborn; the increasing availability of zoster immunoglobulin, however, may allow clinicians to attack the infection before significant fetal viremia has developed. Shingles, which is a reactivation of varicella, would not likely have fetal effects because of already existing maternal IgG from the initial exposure. Herpesvirus can be acquired by the fetus as it passes down the genital tract and can cause a severe, often fatal herpes infection in the newborn.

99. The answer is a. *(Gleicher, 3/e, pp 572–574.)* Both viremia and the excretion of virus from the throats of persons infected with rubella occur 5 to 7 days before the appearance of the characteristic maculopapular rash. The importance of this relationship is that by the time a pregnant woman first notes the appearance of a rash on one of her children, she has already been exposed to the disease and may, in fact, be infected. If one member of a family develops rubella, all other members who are susceptible to the disease usually become infected.

100. The answer is c. *(Gleicher, 3/e, pp 647–652.)* Spectinomycin is the treatment of choice for pregnant women who have asymptomatic *Neisseria gonorrhoeae* infections and who are allergic to penicillin. Erythromycin is another drug effective in treating asymptomatic gonorrhea. Although tetracycline also is an effective alternative to penicillin, its use is generally contraindicated in pregnancy. Administration of chloramphenicol is not recommended to treat women, pregnant or not, who have cervical gonorrhea, and the use of ampicillin or penicillin analogs is contraindicated for penicillin-allergic patients.

101. The answer is e. *(Gleicher, 3/e, pp 595–597.)* Immunization in pregnancy often brings about much concern for both patient and physician. Teratogenic concerns regarding the vaccine must be weighed against the potential for harm from the infectious agent. In the case of hepatitis A and B, rabies, tetanus, and varicella, patients may be treated with hyperimmunoglobulin or pooled immune serum globulin. Inactivated bacterial vaccines can be used for cholera, plague, and typhoid as appropriate. Vaccines for measles and mumps are generally considered contraindicated as these are live viruses, although the rubella vaccine, which is known to have been administered inadvertently to over 1000 pregnant women, has never caused a problem and in fact can be used in selected circumstances of exposure.

102. The answer is d. *(Gleicher, 3/e, pp 594–597.)* Inactivated or formalin-killed vaccines such as those for influenza, typhoid fever, tetanus, pertussis, diphtheria toxoid, rabies, poliomyelitis, cholera, plague, and Rocky Mountain spotted fever are probably not hazardous for either the mother or the fetus. Among the live viral vaccines, such as those for measles, mumps, and poliomyelitis, only the rubella vaccine theoretically may retain its teratogenic properties. There is a 5% to 10% risk of fetal infection when the vaccine is administered during the first trimester. However, no cases of congenital rubella syndrome have been reported in this group of patients. Of the commonly administered attenuated live viral vaccines, only polio virus has the ability to spread from a vaccine to susceptible persons in the immediate environment. Therefore, the risk of infection for the pregnant mother who has been exposed to children who have recently been vaccinated for measles, mumps, and rubella is probably minimal.

103. The answer is a. *(Rodeck, pp 851–853.)* Toxoplasmosis, a protozoal infection caused by *Toxoplasma gondii,* can result from ingestion of raw or undercooked meat infected by the organism or from contact with infected cat feces. The French, because their diet includes raw meat, have a high incidence. The incidence of toxoplasmosis in pregnant women is estimated to be 1 in every 150 to 700 pregnancies. Infection early in pregnancy may cause abortion; later in pregnancy, however, the fetus may become infected. A small number of infected infants develop involvement of the central nervous system or the eye; most infants who have the disease, however, escape serious clinical problems.

104. The answer is e. *(Gleicher, 3/e, pp 754–773.)* Following an elevated toxoplasmosis, other, rubella, cytomegalic inclusion disease, and herpes simplex (TORCH) screen, maternal toxoplasmosis-specific IgM titers are the next step in differentiating between primary infection, which could be dangerous to the fetus, and reexposure, which is not. If the specific IgM is positive, then there is a real risk of transplacental passage and fetal exposure. Since IgM does not cross the placenta, documentation of fetal blood IgM would demonstrate fetal infection. Since IgG does cross, fetal blood IgG will not help determine fetal infection. Amniotic fluid levels are unreliable.

105–108. The answers are 105-a, 106-e, 107-b, 108-d. (*Zatuchni, pp 81–88.*) Fetal exposure to an antibiotic depends on many factors such as gestational age, protein binding, lipid solubility, pH, molecular weight, degree of ionization, and concentration gradient. Some antibiotics are even concentrated in the fetal compartment. Tetracycline is contraindicated in all three trimesters. It has been associated with skeletal abnormalities, staining and hypoplasia of budding fetal teeth, bone hypoplasia, and fatal maternal liver decompensation. With prolonged treatment of tuberculosis (TB) in pregnancy, streptomycin has been associated with fetal hearing loss. Its use is restricted to complicated cases of TB. Nitrofurantoins can cause maternal and fetal hemolytic anemia if glucose-6-phosphate dehydrogenase deficiency is present. Chloramphenicol is noted for causing the gray baby syndrome. Infants are unable to properly metabolize the drug, which reaches toxic levels in about 4 days and can lead to neonatal death within 1 to 2 days. Sulfonamides are associated with kernicterus in the newborn. They compete with bilirubin for binding sites on albumin, thereby leaving more bilirubin free for diffusion into tissues. Sulfonamides should be withheld during the last 2 to 6 wk of pregnancy.

109–113. The answers are 109-c, 110-e, 111-a, 112-d, 113-a. (*Scott, 8/e, pp 579–599. Schwartz, 7/e, pp 126, 1902.*) Group A b-hemolytic streptococci can cause puerperal or postoperative pelvic infection. Outbreaks of puerperal fever are still reported on obstetric services, though not at anywhere near the frequency of 50 years ago. When the disease does occur, a point source among the hospital personnel should be suspected. Group B β-hemolytic streptococci, which can also cause puerperal fever, have recently been recognized as a major cause of severe neonatal infection. The organism can be isolated from the cervices of about 5% of all pregnant women; infection of the infant, which can result in sepsis, occurs as the infant passes through the vagina. *Toxoplasma gondii,* a protozoan parasite, is transmitted by flies from cat feces to human food. Thus, humans can become infected by consuming infected meat that is inadequately cooked or by coming in direct contact with feces of an infected cat. Acute toxoplasmosis in a pregnant woman may cause a fulminant fetal infection; infected neonates may be born with microcephaly, intracranial calcification, or other symptoms. An effective attenuated-virus vaccine is available for immunization against rubella. However, its use is generally contraindicated for pregnant women and commonly is associated with development of arthralgia in adults. Rubella syndrome has not been seen in fetuses when mothers are vaccinated and can be considered if a pregnant woman is exposed to the virus.

114–118. The answers are 114-c, 115-e, 116-a, 117-e, 118-b. (*Scott, 8/e, p 81.*) The recommendations concerning immunizations during pregnancy offered by the American College of Obstetricians and Gynecologists are as follows:

1. Administration of influenza vaccine is recommended if the underlying disease is serious.
2. Typhoid immunization is recommended when one travels to an endemic region.
3. Hepatitis A immunization is recommended after exposure or before travel to developing countries.
4. Cholera immunization should be given only to meet travel requirements.
5. Tetanus-diphtheria immunization should be given if a primary series has never been administered or if 10 years has elapsed without the patient receiving a booster.
6. Immunization for poliomyelitis is mandatory during an epidemic but otherwise not recommended.
7. Smallpox immunization is unnecessary since the disease has been eradicated.
8. Immunization for yellow fever is recommended before travel to a high-risk area.
9. Mumps and rubella immunizations are contraindicated.
10. Administration of rabies vaccine is unaffected by pregnancy.

119–122. The answers are 119-b, 120-e, 121-c, 122-a. (*Reece, 2/e, pp 398–401.*) Viral infections during pregnancy are of great concern. The risk to the fetus is greatest during the first trimester. In most instances, congenital infection results from transplacental transmission of the virus during maternal viremia. In addition, perinatal infection may result from acquisition of virus by passage of the infant through a contaminated birth canal. Cytomegalovirus, rubella, and varicella are well established as teratogens. Congenital disease may range from mild symptoms to major congenital defects to asymptomatic disease with late sequelae. Hepatitis B is only rarely transmitted in utero, but usually at the time of birth, and may cause a mild to severe hepatitis in infancy or, more commonly, result in a carrier state. Carriers run the risk of developing cirrhosis or hepatocellular carcinoma later in life. Rubeola is uncommon in pregnancy and has not been associated with any specific anomalies.

123–124. The answers are 123-a, d; 124-b, c, e. *(Avery, 5/e, pp 1139–1146. James, 2/e, pp 527–529.)* Rubella syndrome in the newborn secondary to rubella infection during pregnancy (especially, though not exclusively, during the first trimester) is well known. Although cytomegalovirus infection is less familiar, it is thought to cause congenital anomalies in about 500 newborns every year in the United States. The abnormalities are usually in the central nervous system and include microcephaly, cerebral calcifications, deafness, and other mental and motor disabilities. Although there have been some suggestions that influenza epidemics have led to a subsequent rise in the incidence of childhood leukemia, this relationship has not been established; in fact, there is no proof that influenza is associated with any anomalies. Mumps is relatively common during pregnancy, but prospective studies have failed to show any associated congenital anomalies. AIDs, while vertically transmissible to the fetus, does not have associated specific fetal anomalies.

125. The answer is e. *(Gleicher, 3/e, pp 263–267.)* Chronic alcohol abuse, which can cause liver disease, folate deficiency, and many other disorders in a pregnant woman, also can lead to the development of congenital abnormalities in the child. The chief abnormalities associated with the fetal alcohol syndrome are microcephaly, growth retardation, and cardiac anomalies. Chronic abuse of alcohol may also be associated with an increased incidence of mental retardation in the children of affected women.

126. The answer is c. *(Gleicher, 3/e, pp 160–164.)* Streeter hypothesized that each organ system has a definite time for appearance and differentiation. Consequently, when an insult occurs, it cannot affect or alter a structure that has differentiated earlier or one that does not develop until after the insult is completed. Major heart and circulatory structures are found from 6 to 8 wk postmenstrual age.

127–128. The answers are 127-a, c, e; 128-b, d. (*Reece, 2/e, pp 398–401.*) Tetracycline may cause fetal dental anomalies and inhibition of bone growth if administered during the second and third trimesters, and it is a potential teratogen to first-trimester fetuses. Administration of tetracycline can also cause severe hepatic decompensation in the mother, especially during the third trimester. Chloramphenicol may cause the gray baby syndrome (symptoms of which include vomiting, impaired respiration, hypothermia, and, finally, cardiovascular collapse) in neonates who have received large doses of the drug. No notable adverse effects have been associated with the use of penicillin or ampicillin. Trimethoprim-sulfamethoxazole (Bactrim) should not be used in the third trimester because sulfa drugs can cause kernicterus.

129. The answer is b. (*Gleicher, 3/e, pp 223–233.*) Fetal therapy is not possible for most serious birth defects but has been successful in a limited number of situations. These include (1) the placement of a suprapubic catheter in utero to allow urine to escape into amniotic fluid to protect the lungs and kidneys in obstructive uropathies, (2) the use of maternally administered cardiac medications that pass through the placenta and can convert selected arrhythmias, (3) dexamethasone steroid suppression of the fetal adrenal gland in the adrenogenital syndrome, which prevents external genital masculinization in affected females, and (4) open or endoscopic fetal surgery with fetal laparotomies to correct diaphragmatic hernias. Treatments for hydrocephaly and porencephalic cysts have been unsuccessful, because these are usually part of a larger syndromic anomaly, and these treatments have been abandoned.

130–132. The answers are 130-a, 131-d, 132-c. (*Gleicher, 3/e, pp 199–200.*) There are four key statistical concepts in the evaluation of screening tests. Sensitivity refers to the ability of the test to accurately identify people who are positive for a disorder. Specificity is the opposite, i.e., of all the people who do not have the disorder, what percentage will in fact test negative? Positive and negative predictive values refer to scenarios starting with a positive or negative test, and then ask, given the positive test, what percentage of people would actually have the disease? By and large, epidemiologists and public health questions center around sensitivity and specificity. Commonly, patient and physician concerns start when a patient who tests positive wants to know what the chances are that she really has the disorder.

133–135. 133-b, 134-b, 135-a. (*Gleicher, 3/e, pp 199–200.*) Diagnostic tests give a definitive answer. They are commonly expensive, are generally only performed on a selected proportion of the population because of their expense and intensity, and give a definitive answer. Screening tests are performed generally on the entire population, the focus of these tests is on being cheap and reliable, and their principal goal is to identify a small percentage of the population that needs to go on to further definitive testing. Occasionally, tests such as ultrasound can in fact be both diagnostic and screening tests. One does a screening ultrasound looking for anomalies, or markers of chromosome abnormalities. Sometimes one may find a marker of an abnormality, such as a nuchal translucency, which, in and of itself, is not diagnostic, or sometimes one may find an actual anomaly, which then becomes diagnostic.

MEDICAL, SURGICAL, AND OBSTETRIC COMPLICATIONS OF PREGNANCY

Questions

DIRECTIONS: Each item below contains a question or incomplete statement followed by suggested responses. Select the **one best** response to each question.

136. Which of the following statements about amniotic fluid volume is true?

a. Fetal membranes are the major source of amniotic fluid in the latter half of pregnancy
b. The fetus starts to swallow amniotic fluid in the third trimester
c. Exchange in the fetal respiratory tract is a major determinant of amniotic fluid volume
d. A large component of amniotic fluid is derived from water transport across fetal skin during the first half of gestation

137. Which of the following statements about progesterone production in pregnancy is true?

a. Progesterone production during the last 10 wk of gestation is largely due to the corpus luteum
b. Progesterone production in the first 12 wk of gestation is largely due to the placenta
c. A major substrate for placental progesterone production is maternal cholesterol
d. Progesterone levels fall rapidly with fetal demise
e. Progesterone serves as the principal substrate for fetal fatty acid synthesis

138. During pregnancy a woman needs additional iron to satisfy the demands of the fetus, the placenta, and her own increasing hemoglobin mass. The total antepartum iron need is approximately.

a. 250 mg
b. 800 mg
c. 1350 mg
d. 1900 mg
e. 2500 mg

139. Changes in pregnancy related to maternal calcium include which of the following?

a. A decrease in maternal parathyroid hormone (PTH) level
b. An increase in ionized calcium concentration
c. A decrease in total serum calcium levels
d. A decrease in absorption of calcium from the gut
e. Response to increased thyroid hormone concentration

140. As pregnancy progresses, which of the following hematologic changes occurs?

a. Plasma volume increases proportionally more than red cell volume
b. Red cell volume increases proportionally more than plasma volume
c. Plasma volume increases and red cell volume remains constant
d. Red cell volume decreases and plasma volume remains constant
e. Neither plasma volume nor red cell volume changes

141. A 24-year-old primigravida at 16 wk gestation has a creatinine of 1.5 mg/dL and a blood urea nitrogen (BUN) of 18 mg/dL. Which of the following is true?

a. An increase in creatinine and BUN is expected with increasing fetal growth
b. The values obtained are normal for gestation
c. Further renal function tests should be obtained
d. These values are normal for the first two trimesters of pregnancy, but not the third trimester
e. The patient can improve renal function by resting in the supine position

142. During pregnancy, the renal glomerular filtration rate (GFR) can increase by as much as

a. 10%
b. 25%
c. 50%
d. 75%
e. 100%

143. In normal pregnancy, which of the following hormones levels remain stable?

a. Total thyroxine (T_4)
b. Parathyroid hormone (PTH) in the second and third trimesters
c. Free cortisol
d. Prolactin

144. Maternal metabolic adaptation in pregnancy includes

a. An increase in dietary nitrogen utilization
b. A decrease in daily protein requirements
c. A shift toward utilization of "empty calories" for energy requirements
d. A decrease in concentration of all plasma proteins
e. An increase in maternal serum albumin

145. A placenta that has a chorionic plate smaller than the basal plate is

a. A membranaceous placenta
b. A succenturiate placenta
c. A circumvallate placenta
d. A fenestrated placenta

146. Insulin secretion in pregnancy is increased by

a. Progesterone
b. Estrogen
c. Growth hormone
d. Human chorionic somatomammotropin
e. Prolactin

147. Changes in the respiratory system during pregnancy include

a. Decreased tidal volume
b. Increased residual volume
c. Decreased respiratory minute volume
d. Increased respiratory rate
e. Increased CO_2

148. The management of maternal thyroid disease can be complicated because of effects on both mother and fetus because which of the following crosses the placenta readily?

a. Thyroxine
b. Long-acting thyroid stimulator
c. Thyroid-stimulating hormone
d. Immunoglobulin M (IgM)
e. Prednisone

149. Which of the following laboratory parameters increases during pregnancy?

a. Serum albumin
b. Blood urea nitrogen
c. Creatinine
d. Erythrocyte sedimentation
e. Bicarbonate

150. Which of the following clotting factors would be decreased during normal pregnancy?

a. Factor XI (plasma thromboplastin antecedent)
b. Factor VIII (antihemophilic globulin)
c. Factor XII
d. Factor IX (plasma thromboplastin component, or Christmas factor)
e. Fibrinogen

151. Maternal ureteral dilation during pregnancy is caused by which of the following?

a. Uterine pressure at the symphysis pubis
b. Pressure from the dilated left ovarian vein
c. Progesterone effect
d. Estrogen effect
e. Increased glomerular filtration rate

152. Substances that are normally found in higher concentrations in the maternal blood than in fetal or umbilical cord blood include

a. Immunoglobulin G (IgG)
b. Immunoglobulin M (IgM)
c. γ chains of hemoglobin
d. Threonine
e. Cysteamine β-mercaptoethylamine

153. Which of the following statements concerning abdominal pregnancy is correct?

a. Gastrointestinal symptoms are quite often severe
b. Fetal survival is approximately 50%
c. Aggressive attempts should be made to remove the placenta at the time of initial surgery
d. It may result in infectious morbidity prior to the diagnosis
e. It is usually the result of a primary abdominal implantation

154. The adult respiratory distress syndrome can be seen during pregnancy in association with

a. Increased airway pressure
b. Increased functional residual capacity
c. Increased lung compliance
d. An early proliferative phase with type I cell proliferation
e. A late exudative phase with type II cell destruction

155. Which of the following statements about placental abruption is true?

a. Coagulopathy results from the consumption of clotting factors by the retroplacental clot
b. More than 50% of patients with this condition develop significant hypofibrinogenemia (less than 150 mg/dL)
c. Less than 10% of patients with this condition develop significant hypofibrinogenemia (less than 150 mg/dL)
d. Vigorous fluid, blood, and electrolyte replacement is generally adequate to prevent severe renal failure
e. Many patients require dialysis despite vigorous fluid, blood, and electrolyte replacement

156. Which of the following statements concerning placenta previa is true?

a. Its incidence decreases with maternal age
b. Its incidence is unaffected by parity
c. The initial hemorrhage is usually painless and rarely fatal
d. Management no longer includes a double setup
e. Vaginal examination should be done immediately upon suspicion of placenta previa

157. For patients who develop preeclampsia in their first pregnancy, which of the following is an associated future risk?

a. Diabetes mellitus
b. Chronic hypertension
c. Habitual abortion
d. Chronic liver disease
e. Increased risk of third-trimester stillborns in subsequent pregnancies

158. A patient at 17 wk gestation is diagnosed as having an intrauterine fetal demise. She returns to your office 5 wk later and has not had a miscarriage, although she has had some occasional spotting. This patient is at increased risk for

a. Septic abortion
b. Recurrent abortion
c. Consumptive coagulopathy with hypofibrinogenemia
d. Future infertility
e. Ectopic pregnancies

159. Which of the following statements concerning appendicitis in pregnancy is true?

a. Diagnosis is similar to that in the nonpregnant patient
b. The maternal death rate is highest in the first trimester
c. Surgical treatment should be delayed until the diagnosis is firmly established
d. The incidence is unchanged by pregnancy
e. The rate of fetal loss is about 50%

160. Which of the following statements concerning hepatitis infection in pregnancy is true?

a. Hepatitis B core antigen status is the most sensitive indicator of positive vertical transmission of disease
b. Hepatitis B is the most common form of hepatitis after blood transfusion
c. The proper treatment of infants born to infected mothers includes the administration of hepatitis B immune globulin as well as Heptavax-B
d. Patients who develop chronic active hepatitis should undergo therapeutic abortion

161. A 24-year-old woman appears at 8 wk of pregnancy and reveals a history of pulmonary embolism 7 years ago during her first pregnancy. She was treated with intravenous heparin followed by several months of oral warfarin (Coumadin) and has had no further evidence of thromboembolic disease for over 6 years. Which of the following statements about her current condition is true?

a. Having no evidence of disease for over 5 years means that the risk of thromboembolism is not greater than normal
b. Impedance plethysmography is not a useful study to evaluate her for deep venous thrombosis in pregnancy
c. Doppler ultrasonography is not a useful technique to evaluate her for deep venous thrombosis in pregnancy
d. The patient should be placed on low-dose heparin therapy throughout pregnancy and puerperium
e. The patient is at highest risk for recurrent thromboembolism during the second trimester of pregnancy

162. Which of the following statements concerning urinary tract infection in pregnancy is true?

a. In cases of acute pyelonephritis, the most common organism cultured is group B streptococcus
b. Women with sickle cell trait possess a protective mechanism against urinary tract infections, and they have an overall lower incidence of bacteriuria during pregnancy
c. Culture of a clean-voided midstream urine specimen is adequate for the diagnosis of asymptomatic bacteriuria (ASB)
d. Because as many as 40% of women with asymptomatic bacteriuria may progress to symptomatic disease, intravenous antibiotic therapy should be instituted once the diagnosis is made
e. Asymptomatic bacteriuria affects 20% of pregnancies

163. The most common pathogen causing urinary tract infection (UTI) in pregnancy is

a. *Pseudomonas aeruginos*
b. *Proteus mirabilis*
c. *Haemophilus influenzae*
d. *Escherichia coli*
e. *Klebsiella pneumoniae*

164. A 29-year-old, gravida 3, para 2 black woman in the 33d wk of gestation is admitted to the emergency room because of acute abdominal pain that developed and is increasing during the past 24 h. The pain is severe and is radiating from the epigastrium to the back. The patient has vomited a few times and has not eaten or had a bowel movement since the pain started. On examination you observe an acutely ill patient lying on the bed with her knees drawn up. Her blood pressure is 150/100 mm Hg, her pulse is 110 beats/min, and her temperature is 38.18°C (100.68°F). On palpation the abdomen is somewhat distended and tender, mainly in the epigastric area, and the uterine fundus reaches 31 cm above the symphysis. Hypotonic bowel sounds are noted. Fetal monitoring reveals a normal pattern of fetal heart rate (FHR) without uterine contractions. On ultrasonography the fetus is in vertex presentation and appropriate in size for gestational age; fetal breathing and trunk movements are noted and the volume of amniotic fluid is normal. The placenta is located on the anterior uterine wall and of grade 2 to 3. Laboratory values show mild leukocytosis (12,000 cells/µL); a hematocrit of 43; mildly elevated serum glutamic-oxaloacetic transaminase (SGOT), serum glutamic-pyruvic transaminase (SGPT), and bilirubin; and serum amylase of 180 U/dL. Urinalysis is normal.

The most probable diagnosis in this patient is

a. Acute degeneration of uterine leiomyoma
b. Acute cholecystitis
c. Acute pancreatitis
d. Acute appendicitis
e. Severe preeclamptic toxemia

165. Although rheumatic heart disease is less common than in previous decades, it still occurs during pregnancy. Deteriorating cardiac status in a pregnant woman is most likely to be associated with

a. Aortic regurgitation
b. Aortic stenosis
c. Mitral regurgitation
d. Mitral stenosis
e. Tricuspid regurgitation

166. An 18-year-old has asymptomatic bacteriuria at her first prenatal visit at 15 wk gestation. Which of the following statements is true?

a. The prevalence of ASB during pregnancy may be as great as 30%
b. There is a decreased incidence of ASB in multiparas with sickle cell trait
c. 15% of women develop a urinary tract infection after an initial negative urine culture
d. 10% of women with ASB subsequently develop an acute symptomatic urinary infection during that pregnancy
e. 1% of women with ASB have pyelographic evidence of chronic infection or congenital abnormalities of the urinary tract

167. When treating urinary tract infection (UTI) in the third trimester, the antibiotic of choice should be

a. Cephalosporin
b. Tetracycline
c. Sulfonamide
d. Nitrofurantoin

168. Which of the following statements about autoimmune thrombocytopenic purpura (ATP) in pregnancy are true?

a. Platelet production is depressed in the bone marrow
b. Bleeding time may be normal because of the presence in the circulation of young, hyperactive platelets
c. Peripheral destruction of antibody-coated circulating platelets may result in abnormally low maternal platelet counts
d. Cesarean section always prevents fetal hemorrhage
e. A maternal platelet count above 10,000/μL at the time of delivery ensures safety for the newborn

169. A 24-year-old presents at 30 wk with a 50-cm fundal height. Which of the following statements concerning polyhydramnios is true?

a. Acute polyhydramnios always leads to labor prior to 28 wk
b. The incidence of associated malformations is approximately 3%
c. Maternal edema, especially of the lower extremities and vulva, is rare
d. Esophageal atresia is accompanied by polyhydramnios in nearly 10% of cases
e. Complications include placental abruption, uterine dysfunction, and postpartum hemorrhage

170. True statements about acquired immune deficiency syndrome (AIDS) in pregnancy include

a. *Pneumocystis carinii* pneumonia is the most common opportunistic infection
b. Women tolerate AIDS better than men
c. Genital herpes in pregnancy is protective against AIDS
d. Vertical transmission is the most common method of infection with AIDS
e. Breast feeding is safe for AIDS-positive mothers

171. True statements about pregnancy-induced hypertension include which of the following?

a. The incidence varies little around the world
b. Women who have had hypertension of pregnancy once have a 10% chance of developing it in a later pregnancy
c. Elevations in systolic or diastolic blood pressures do not become diagnostically significant until blood pressure values reach 140/90 mm Hg
d. Young primiparous women have the lowest incidence
e. Having a baby by a different father increases the risk of preeclampsia in a multigravid woman

172. Pregnancy has which of the following effects on diabetic women?

a. Tendency toward ketoacidosis during early pregnancy
b. Tendency toward hyperglycemia during early pregnancy
c. Increase in insulin requirement during early pregnancy
d. Reduction of placental transfer of glucose by hyperglycemia
e. Increase in insulin requirement during late pregnancy

173. A 30-year-old class D diabetic is concerned about pregnancy. She can be assured that which of the following risks is the same for her as for the general population?

a. Preeclampsia and eclampsia
b. Infection
c. Fetal cystic fibrosis
d. Postpartum hemorrhage after vaginal delivery
e. Hydramnios

174. Systemic lupus erythematosus (SLE) in pregnancy

a. Has a similar incidence among ethnic groups
b. Is likely to worsen if the patient was in remission before pregnancy
c. May be associated with a syndrome of thrombocytopenia in pregnancy
d. May cause more wastage of male fetuses
e. Has a lower incidence of preeclampsia-like syndrome (hypertension, proteinuria)

175. For a diabetic patient, which of the following is safest for the fetus?

a. Glycosuria
b. Ketoacidosis
c. Ketonuria in the absence of diabetic ketoacidosis
d. Hyperglycemia
e. Hypoglycemia

176. True statements regarding the interaction between maternal epilepsy and pregnancy include which of the following?

a. Seizure frequency increases in about 90% of epileptic mothers during pregnancy
b. When seizure frequency increases, it most commonly does so during the third trimester or immediately postpartum
c. Epileptic women have a significant risk of stillbirth
d. Breast feeding in epileptic women should be discouraged because of neonatal effects of antiepileptic drugs secreted in milk
e. Phenytoin (Dilantin) therapy decreases the risk of epilepsy-related congenital malformations

177. Which of the following is the same for hyperthyroid and euthyroid pregnant women?

a. Response to thiourea compounds
b. Concentration of long-acting thyroid stimulator (LATS)
c. Incidence of neonatal thyrotoxicosis
d. Indications for interrupting a pregnancy
e. Thyroid functions postpartum

178. Which of the following statements about hypothyroidism in pregnancy is true?

a. It is common during pregnancy
b. It is not associated with an increased abortion rate
c. It is not associated with an increased stillbirth rate
d. It is generally improved by pregnancy
e. It can cause fetal hypothyroidism

179. A 37-year-old, G4, P3 woman has erythroblastosis fetalis. Which of the following is least likely to be related?

a. Kell blood group
b. Kidd blood group
c. Duffy blood group
d. Lewis blood group
e. ABO blood group

180. True statements about the twin-twin transfusion syndrome include which of the following?

a. The donor twin develops hydramnios more often than does the recipient twin
b. Gross differences may be observed between donor and recipient placentas
c. The donor twin usually suffers from a hemolytic anemia
d. The donor twin is more likely to develop widespread thromboses
e. The donor twin often develops polycythemia

181. A 32-year-old, G3, P0, spontaneous abortion × 3 woman has just had her third loss between 20 and 24 wk. Which of the following is mostly likely to be the same for this patient as for women without such losses?

a. Painless dilatation of the cervix
b. History of cervical trauma
c. Spontaneous rupture of the membranes at midpregnancy
d. History of previous induced abortions
e. Recurrent losses at 25 to 27 wk gestation

182. You are called in to evaluate the heart of a 19-year-old primigravida at term. Listening carefully to the heart, you determine that there is a split S_1, normal S_2, S_3 easily audible with a 2/6 systolic ejection murmur greater during inspiration, and a soft diastolic murmur. You immediately recognize that

a. The presence of the S_3 is abnormal
b. The systolic ejection murmur is unusual in a pregnant woman at term
c. Diastolic murmurs are rare in a pregnant woman
d. The combination of a prominent S_3 and soft diastolic murmur is a significant abnormality
e. All findings recorded are normal changes in pregnancy

183. Pregnancy should be strongly discouraged in women who have

a. Atrial septal defect
b. Ventricular septal defect
c. Patent ductus arteriosus
d. Eisenmenger syndrome
e. Wolff-Parkinson-White arrhythmia

184. A 30-year-old has quadruplets following in vitro fertilization (IVF). In counseling her, you can reassure her that which of the following has the lowest impact on the outcome of reduction?

a. Technique of induction of ovulation
b. Starting number
c. Finishing number
d. Gestational age at procedure
e. Operator experience

185. A 21-year-old has a positive purified protein derivative (PPD) and is about to be treated for tuberculosis. She can be reassured that which of the following is minimal?

a. Rifampin may cause a flulike syndrome
b. Patients receiving isoniazid (INH) may develop a peripheral neuropathy
c. Patients receiving INH may develop optic neuritis
d. Ototoxicity is a side effect of streptomycin
e. A positive antinuclear antibody (ANA) titer may be seen with INH therapy

186. The use of aspirin in pregnancy may be associated with which of the following complications?

a. Oligohydramnios
b. Polyhydramnios
c. Fetal platelet dysfunction
d. Premature labor
e. Neonatal jaundice

187. Which of the following is consistent with a decision to perform a cerclage?

a. Uterine contractions
b. Cervix dilated to 3 cm
c. Uterine bleeding
d. Gestation of 26 wk
e. Chorioamnionitis

MEDICAL, SURGICAL, AND OBSTETRIC COMPLICATIONS OF PREGNANCY

Answers

136. The answer is d. (*Gleicher, 3/e, pp 65–66.*) There are three major determinants of amniotic fluid volume throughout gestation: (1) movement of water and solutes across fetal membranes, (2) fetal physiologic regulation of flow rates, such as urine production and swallowing, and (3) maternal effects on transplacental fluid movement. Fetal urine is a major source of amniotic fluid in the second half of gestation, as proved by the anhydramnios associated with Potter syndrome (renal agenesis) or with urinary tract obstruction. The fetus begins to swallow amniotic fluid at 8 to 11 wk of gestation; obstruction of the gastrointestinal (GI) tract (e.g., esophageal atresia) is associated with polyhydramnios in most cases. During the first half of pregnancy, it is likely that a large component of amniotic fluid is derived from water transport across the highly permeable skin of the fetus. Even though it is obvious that amniotic fluid is important for the development of the fetal respiratory tract, it is unclear whether the outflow of lung fluid contributes to amniotic fluid volume. Animal studies suggest that such an outflow of lung fluid occurs, but that fluid is swallowed before it enters the amniotic space.

137. The answer is c. (*Gleicher, 3/e, pp 119, 233–234, 276.*) The corpus luteum constitutes the major source of progesterone production during the first 10 wk of pregnancy. The placenta represents the major source of progesterone production after the first 12 wk. As the placenta is unable to synthesize cholesterol from acetate, the major substrate for placental progesterone production comes from maternal cholesterol. Fetal synthesis of progesterone contributes little to the maternal levels; therefore, progesterone levels will remain high even after fetal demise. The most important role of progesterone in the fetus is as a substrate for fetal adrenal gland production of glucocorticoids and mineralocorticoids.

138. The answer is b. (*Gleicher, 3/e, pp 316–317, 1156.*) The fetus and placenta contain approximately 300 mg of elemental iron at birth. In addition, the maternal increase in hemoglobin mass accounts for about 500 mg of elemental iron. Thus, the total antepartum iron requirement is 800 mg. Most of this iron is needed during the second half of pregnancy, at an approximate rate of 5.7 mg daily during the last 140 days. However, because about 1 mg of iron is excreted daily, the total daily iron need is almost 7 mg during the second half of pregnancy. Most women of childbearing age cannot mobilize this much iron, and supplemental iron must be given to prevent iron deficiency. The usual iron supplement, ferrous sulfate, contains 20% elemental iron. Thus, a 325-mg tablet contains about 65 mg of elemental iron, of which 10% to 20% will be absorbed. Most prenatal vitamins contain 60 or 65 mg of iron, and these should be adequate for a healthy pregnant woman. If iron stores have been depleted by poor dietary habits, recent childbirth, or other causes, however, additional iron supplementation may be necessary.

139. The answer is c. (*Gleicher, 3/e, pp 1372–1373, 1551–1560.*) Levels of maternal total serum calcium decline throughout pregnancy until 34 to 36 gestational weeks, paralleling the fall in concentration of maternal serum albumin. The concentration of maternal serum ionized calcium is constant throughout pregnancy and unchanged from values in nonpregnant women. The constant concentration of ionized calcium despite the pregnancy-specific changes in plasma volume and glomerular filtration rate (GFR) is attributable to a marked increase in PTH in pregnancy, which causes increased absorption of calcium from the gut and decreased renal loss of calcium. The skeleton is maintained during this "physiologic hyperparathyroidism" by the action of calcitonin, and is independent of thyroid status.

140. The answer is a. (*Reece, 2/e, p 905.*) During pregnancy, the plasma volume increases by about 48% and the red cell volume increases by about 30%. The rapid increase in the plasma volume occurs during early pregnancy, while the red cell volume rises more rapidly after the first trimester of pregnancy. As a result, hematocrit values during the first trimester and most of the second trimester of pregnancy could be much lower than normal. The reduction in hematocrit constitutes the "physiologic anemia" of pregnancy.

141. The answer is c. *(Gleicher, 3/e, p 998.)* In pregnancy the glomerular filtration rate (GFR) increases by as much as 50%. This increase in GFR produces a relative decrease in creatinine and BUN. Further tests of renal function, such as creatinine clearance, should be performed to evaluate renal function in this patient. Renal function is improved in a lateral recumbent position.

142. The answer is c. *(Gleicher, 3/e, p 998.)* The glomerular filtration rate (GFR) increases early in pregnancy—by as much as 50% by the beginning of the second trimester. The elevated GFR persists to term. The precise mechanism has not been identified.

143. The answer is c. *(Gleicher, 3/e, pp 433–434.)* During pregnancy there is moderate hyperplasia of the thyroid gland, resulting in a sharp increase in thyroxine (T_4) concentration noted already in the 2nd mo. However, owing to a concomitant increase in thyroxine-binding globulins (TBGs) in maternal plasma, the amount of free, biologically active T_4 is not changed significantly. Plasma PTH concentration decreases in the first trimester but increases progressively throughout the rest of gestation. Estrogens appear to block the effect of PTH on bone resorption; it seems that during pregnancy a new set point exists between ionized calcium and PTH. Prolactin levels increase constantly throughout gestation; the mean level of prolactin at term is about 10 times higher than in the nonpregnant state. Circulating cortisol also increases considerably, but most of it is bound to transcortin and free cortisol levels are not elevated. The rate of cortisol secretion by the maternal adrenal is not increased (and probably is somewhat decreased) compared with adrenal activity in nonpregnant women. The increase in circulating cortisol is the result of the decreased metabolic clearance rate of cortisol in pregnancy.

144. The answer is c. *(Gleicher, 3/e, pp 25–32.)* The products of conception are relatively rich in protein—at term the fetus and placenta contain approximately 500 g of protein, about one-half of the total increase in pregnancy. The remaining 500 g of protein are added to the mother's uterus, breasts, and blood (in the form of Hg and plasma proteins). Since dietary nitrogen utilization during pregnancy is only 26% of prepregnancy values, daily protein requirements are increased significantly to supply increased demands despite decreased utilization. For maximal protein utilization, maternal energy requirements should be met by adequate fat and carbohydrate intake. With increasing intake of fat and carbohydrates as energy sources, less dietary protein is required to maintain a positive nitrogen balance. Plasma protein concentrations may be altered in pregnancy. Albumin concentration decreases and fibrinogen, transferrin, ceruloplasmin, and α_1 antitrypsin increase with advancing gestation. Complement C2 and haptoglobin concentration are apparently not changed in pregnancy.

145. The answer is c. *(Gleicher, 3/e, pp 352–355.)* Abnormalities of placentation in which the chorionic plate is smaller than the basal plate include circumvallate and circummarginate placentas; these are known as extrachorial placentas. Succenturiate placentas have accessory lobes in the membrane away from the main body of the placenta; these lobes are connected by large vessels to the main body. A membranaceous placenta has functioning villi covering all the fetal membranes, and a fenestrated placenta is one in which the central portion of the placenta is missing.

146. The answer is d. *(Rodeck, pp 112–114.)* The tendency for pregnancy to be diabetogenic is thought to be mainly due to the anti-insulin effects of many of the hormones secreted by the placenta as well as to the possible effect of insulin receptors on the placenta itself. Human chorionic somatomammotropin (also known as human placental lactogen) is present in large amounts in the maternal circulation during the third trimester. Its lipolytic and other actions inhibit glucose uptake and manufacture and therefore stimulate insulin production to rise. Levels of pituitary growth hormone are decreased, especially during late pregnancy, and probably have little to do with increased insulin needs. Prolactin rises in the third trimester but is independent of insulin requirements. Estrogen and progesterone, both of which are present in increased amounts during pregnancy, probably act as peripheral insulin antagonists and therefore would lead to decreased insulin utilization.

147. The answer is d. *(Reece, 2/e, pp 911.)* Progesterone is thought to result in gradually increasing tidal volume (volume of air moved) to 30% to 40% above baseline at term. Consequently, the residual volume is decreased with increased respiratory minute volume. Although respiratory rate remains unchanged, the increased respiratory minute volume causes a decrease in

CO_2 in the alveoli and blood, which results in the "hyperventilation" of the pregnancy.

148. The answer is b. *(Reece, 2/e, pp 875–876.)* Thyroxine crosses the placenta poorly if at all. For this reason a hyperthyroid mother does not transmit her hyperthyroidism to the fetus, and giving thyroid hormone to a hypothyroid mother will not raise fetal thyroxine levels significantly. Propylthiouracil (PTU), an antithyroid drug, crosses easily and may suppress fetal thyroid function. Hyperthyroid women taking large doses of PTU therefore run the risk of having goitrous babies. Some clinicians, hoping to reverse the effect of PTU on the fetus, have given thyroxine to the mother; theoretically, however, this should not work because the thyroid hormone should not get to the fetus. Long-acting thyroid stimulator (LATS) is present in many patients who have Graves' disease. Because LATS can cross the placenta, LATS levels should be obtained from such patients and the pediatrician should be alerted to possible neonatal thyrotoxicosis if LATS is present.

149. The answer is d. *(Reece, 2/e, pp 905–907.)* Plasma fibrinogen levels increase by about 50% during pregnancy. This rise is thought to be at least partially responsible for the great increase in the erythrocyte sedimentation rate. The elevated sedimentation rate is consequently almost useless as a significant laboratory value in pregnant women. Serum albumin decreases by about 30% during normal pregnancy. Blood urea nitrogen (BUN) and creatinine decrease markedly during pregnancy; in fact, BUN values falling in the middle of the normal range for nonpregnant women (i.e., around 10 mg/dL) may signal significant impairment of renal function in pregnant women. P_{CO_2} and bicarbonate decrease secondary to respiratory rate and tidal volume changes.

150. The answer is a. *(Reece, 2/e, pp 908–910.)* There are numerous changes that occur in the coagulation factors during normal pregnancy. Plasma fibrinogen increases approximately 50%, with a corresponding increase in sedimentation rate in pregnancy. Other factors increasing significantly during pregnancy include factor VII, factor VIII, factor IX, and factor X. Factor II (prothrombin) is increased only slightly. Factor XI and factor XIII decrease slightly during pregnancy. The platelet count may decrease slightly during pregnancy. Prothrombin time (PT) and partial thromboplastin time (PTT) are slightly decreased; however, clotting time remains unchanged.

151. The answer is c. *(Reece, 2/e, pp 911.)* One of the common areas of ureteral compression is at the pelvic brim. As the uterus rises out of the pelvis, it compresses the ureters at the pelvic brim. The right ureter seems to be dilated more than the left ureter, and it is thought that the dilated right ovarian vein contributes to the pressure on the right. Progesterone, but not estrogen, is a smooth muscle relaxant and may contribute to the presence of the hydroureters. An increased glomerular filtration rate would not cause the ureters to dilate.

152. The answer is b. *(Cunningham 20/e, pp 159, 163, 168.)* Immunoglobulin G (IgG) easily crosses the placenta and thus is found in approximately equal amounts in maternal and fetal blood. Immunoglobulin M (IgM), on the other hand, is a large molecule and does not cross the placenta. Thus maternal levels of IgM are higher than fetal levels, unless an intrauterine infection causes the fetus to manufacture IgM. The gamma chains in hemoglobin (Hb) are what distinguish fetal hemoglobin from adult hemoglobin. Fetal hemoglobin (Hb F) contains two α and two γ chains. Hb A, found in most adults, contains two α and two β chains. One would therefore expect to find more γ chains in the fetal blood than in maternal blood. All amino acids except glutamine are actively transferred to the fetus and have higher fetal concentrations.

153. The answer is d. *(Schwartz, 7/e, pp 1838–43. Ransom 2000, p 36–37.)* Abdominal pregnancy usually follows a tubal pregnancy with either tubal rupture or spontaneous passage through the fimbriated end. Although women with abdominal pregnancy usually report an increase in gastrointestinal symptoms, these are rarely severe enough to lead to investigation. Fetal death rates are reported to be above 90% with abdominal pregnancies. Infection of the gestational products can occur especially when the placenta adheres to the intestines. This can lead to abscess formation and the possibility of rupture. Although leaving the placenta in the abdomen following surgical delivery predisposes to postoperative coagulation problems as well as the need for subsequent surgery, these complications can be less severe than the hemorrhage associated with attempts at removal at the time of primary delivery. If the placenta cannot easily be removed, recommendations are to leave it in place at the time of the first surgery.

154. The answer is a. *(Reece, 2/e, pp 1691–1693.)* The adult respiratory distress syndrome is an acute injury to the lung that results in marked intrapulmonary shunting and decreased lung compliance. Airway pressure is increased. Residual capacity decreases. There is an early exudative phase characterized by type I cell destruction. Later, atelectasis and neutrophil infiltration lead to a proliferative phase with type II cell proliferation. The overall mortality is 50% to 70%. Treatment is based upon the underlying etiology. For example, treating infection with antibiotics as appropriate, instituting supportive therapy for renal and cardiac symptoms, maintaining proper oxygenation and mechanical ventilation if necessary, along with positive end-expiratory pressure, and normalizing the acid-base status are central to effective therapy.

155. The answer is d. *(Reece, 2/e pp 897–898, 1489.)* Thirty percent of abruptions resulting in fetal death also result in significant hypofibrinogenemia. The mechanism of the coagulopathy is most likely not just the consumption of clotting factors by the retroplacental clot, but rather a disseminated intravascular coagulation. When severe hemorrhage occurs, there is definite risk of acute renal failure. This complication can be prevented through vigorous fluid, blood, and electrolyte replacement, thereby avoiding the need for dialysis.

156. The answer is c. *(Reece, 2/e, 975–976, 1197, 1201.)* The initial hemorrhage in placenta previa is usually painless and rarely fatal. If the fetus is premature and if hemorrhaging is not severe, vaginal examination of a woman suspected of having placenta previa frequently can be delayed until 37 wk of gestation; this delay in the potentially hazardous examination reduces the risk of prematurity, which often is associated with placenta previa. Vaginal examination, when needed to determine whether a low-lying placenta is covering the internal os of the cervix, should be performed in an operating room fully prepared for an emergency cesarean section (i.e., a double setup). Increasing maternal age and multiparity are associated with a higher incidence of placenta previa.

157. The answer is a. *(Gleicher, 3/e, pp 1035–1040.)* Careful long-term follow-up studies of preeclamptic women have failed to reveal long-term hypertensive disease. However, Chesley and colleagues showed diabetes to be 2.5 to 4 times more common in previously preeclamptic women than in controls. When patients with chronic hypertension are removed from these studies, pure preeclampsia seems to have little other long-term risk.

158. The answer is c. *(Gleicher, 3/e, p 1153.)* In modern clinical medicine, once the diagnosis of fetal demise has been made, the products of conception are removed. If, however, the gestational age was over 14 wk and the fetal death occurred 5 wk ago, coagulation abnormalities could be seen. Septic abortions were more frequently seen during the era of illegal abortions, although occasionally sepsis can occur if there is incomplete evacuation of the products of conception in either a therapeutic or spontaneous abortion.

159. The answer is d. *(Gleicher, 3/e, pp 1512–1515.)* The incidence of appendicitis in pregnancy is 1:2000, unchanged from that of the nonpregnant population. The diagnosis is very difficult in pregnancy because leukocytosis, nausea, and vomiting are common in pregnancy and the upward displacement of the appendix by the uterus may cause appendicitis to simulate cholecystitis, pyelonephritis, gastritis, or degenerating myomata. Surgery is necessary even if the diagnosis is not certain. Delays in surgery due to difficulty in diagnosis as the appendix moves up are probably the cause of an increasing maternal mortality with increasing gestational age. Premature birth and abortion account for a rate of fetal loss close to 15%.

160. The answer is c. *(James, 2/e, pp 540–543.)* Persons at increased risk for hepatitis B infection include homosexuals, abusers of intravenous drugs, health care personnel, and people who have received blood or blood products. Also, hepatitis B is endemic in some populations of Asia and Africa. The mode of transmission for hepatitis B is through blood and blood products, as well as saliva, vaginal secretions, and semen. However, because of intensive screening of blood for type B hepatitis, non-A, non-B hepatitis has become the major form of hepatitis after blood transfusion. Venereal transmission and the sharing of needles in persons who abuse intravenous drugs have had major roles in the transmission of hepatitis B. A variety of immunologic markers exist to identify patients who either have active disease, are chronic carriers of disease, or have antibody protection. Among the markers, the e antigen is very similar to the virus and is an indicator of the infectious state. Mothers who are e antigen positive are more likely to transmit the disease to their infants, whereas the absence of the e antigen in the presence of e antibody appears to be protective. Chronic acute hepatitis does not necessarily warrant therapeutic abortion. Fertility is decreased, but pregnancy may proceed on a normal course, as long as steroid therapy is continued. Prematurity and fetal loss are increased, but there is no increase in malformations.

161. The answer is d. *(Gleicher, 3/e, pp 1540–1541.)* Patients with a history of thromboembolic disease in pregnancy are at high risk to develop it in subsequent pregnancies. Impedance plethysmography and Doppler ultrasonography are useful techniques even in pregnancy and should be done as baseline studies. Patients should be treated prophylactically with low-dose heparin therapy through the postpartum period as this is the time of highest risk of this disease.

162. The answer is c. *(Reece, 2/e, pp 1277–1280.)* Asymptomatic bacteriuria is present in approximately 5% of all pregnant women at their first prenatal visit. The overall incidence varies between 2% and 12%, depending on the patient population. The highest incidence appears to be in black multiparous women of low socioeconomic status who have sickle cell trait. Significant bacteriuria is required for diagnosis, which is accomplished by culturing a clean-catch, midstream, voided specimen and demonstrating positive bacterial growth. This avoids routine catheterization with its subsequent increased risk of infection. Twenty to forty percent of women with asymptomatic bacteriuria will progress to a symptomatic infection. Therefore, treatment should be initiated after the diagnosis is made. However, outpatient oral management is appropriate with asymptomatic or symptomatic bacteriuria of the lower urinary tract.

163. The answer is d. *(Reece, 2/e, pp 1277–1280.)* *Escherichia coli* is the most common pathogen to infect the urinary tract in pregnancy. It is responsible for 75% to 90% of bacteriuria in pregnancy and for 70% of cases of acute pyelonephritis. Although more common as a cause of pyelonephritis than of bacteriuria in pregnancy, pseudomonas and proteus are the pathogens in only 5% to 10% of those cases. The parenchymal infection caused by pseudomonas or proteus, however, may be more difficult to eradicate. *Haemophilus influenzae* is a rare cause of UTI in pregnancy, although it is quite commonly an inhabitant of the lower genital tract.

164. The answer is c. *(Reece, 2/e, pp 1142–1145.)* The most probable diagnosis in this case is acute pancreatitis. The pain caused by a myoma in degeneration is more localized to the uterine wall. Low-grade fever and mild leukocytosis may appear with a degenerating myoma, but liver function tests are usually normal. The other obstetric cause of epigastric pain, severe preeclamptic toxemia (PET), may exhibit disturbed liver function [sometimes associated with the HELLP syndrome (hemolysis, elevated liver enzymes, low platelets)], but this patient has only mild elevation of blood pressure and no proteinuria. Acute appendicitis in pregnancy is one of the more common nonobstetric causes of abdominal pain. In pregnancy symptoms of acute appendicitis are similar to those in nonpregnant patients, but the pain is more vague and poorly localized and the point of maximal tenderness moves with advancing gestation to the right upper quadrant. Liver function tests are normal with acute appendicitis. Acute cholecystitis may cause fever, leukocytosis, and pain of the right upper quadrant with abnormal liver function tests, but amylase levels would be elevated only mildly, if at all, and pain would be less severe than described in this patient. The diagnosis that fits the clinical description and the laboratory findings is acute pancreatitis. This disorder may be more common during pregnancy, with an incidence of 1:100 to 1:10,000 pregnancies. Cholelithiasis, chronic alcoholism, infection, abdominal trauma, some medications, and pregnancy-induced hypertension are known predisposing factors. Patients with pancreatitis are usually in acute distress—the classic finding is a person who is rocking with knees drawn up and trunk flexed in agony. Fever, tachypnea, hypotension, ascites, and pleural effusion may be observed. Hypotonic bowel sounds, epigastric tenderness, and signs of peritonitis may be demonstrated on examination.

Leukocytosis, hemoconcentration, and abnormal liver function tests are common laboratory findings in acute pancreatitis. The most important laboratory finding is, however, an elevation of serum amylase levels, which appears 12 to 24 h after onset of clinical disease. Values may exceed 200 U/dL (normal values are 50 to 160 U/dL). A useful diagnostic tool in the pregnant patient with only modest elevation of amylase values is the amylase/creatinine ratio. In patients with acute pancreatitis, the ratio of amylase clearance to creatinine clearance is always greater than 5% to 6%.

Treatment considerations for the pregnant patient with acute pancreatitis are similar to those in nonpregnant patients. Intravenous hydration, nasogastric suction, enteric rest, and correction of electrolyte imbalance and of hyperglycemia are the mainstays of therapy. Careful attention to tissue perfusion, volume expansion, and transfusions to maintain a stable cardiovascular performance are critical. Gradual recovery occurs over 5 to 6 days.

165. The answer is d. *(Reece, 2/e, pp 1026–1027.)* Nearly all the circulatory changes that normally accompany pregnancy are harmful to a woman who has mitral stenosis. Left atrial pressure rises because of increased cardiac output and shortened diastolic filling time; as a result, pulmonary flow is accentuated. Atrial fibrillation may occur suddenly during pregnancy, and pulmonary edema may supervene. Cardioversion may be necessary to reverse atrial fibrillation. Mitral regurgitation is unlikely to be worsened by pregnancy, although prophylaxis for subacute bacterial endocarditis would be indicated for affected women. Aortic stenosis is unusual as a pure lesion; associated problems, if they are going to develop at all, are most likely to develop in the immediate postpartum period, when rapid volume shifts can occur. Aortic regurgitation also is rare as a pure lesion and again is most likely to cause problems just after delivery.

166. The answer is d. *(Reece, 2/e, pp 1277–1280.)* The term *asymptomatic bacteriuria* is used to indicate persisting, actively multiplying bacteria within the urinary tract without symptoms of a urinary infection. The reported prevalence during pregnancy varies from 2% to as great as 12%. The highest incidence has been reported in black multiparas with sickle cell trait. In women who demonstrate ASB, the bacteriuria is typically present at the time of the first prenatal visit; after an initial negative culture of the urine, fewer than 1.5% acquire a urinary infection. Twenty to forty percent of women with ASB develop an acute infection during that pregnancy. Postpartum urologic investigation has often shown pyelographic evidence of chronic infection, obstructive lesions, or congenital abnormalities of the urinary tract.

167. The answer is a. *(Reece, 2/e, pp 1277–1280.)* Although quite effective, sulfonamides should be avoided during the last few weeks of pregnancy because they competitively inhibit the binding of bilirubin to albumin, which increases the risk of neonatal hyperbilirubinemia. Nitrofurantoin may not be tolerated in pregnancy because of the effect of nausea. It should also be avoided in late pregnancy because of the risk of hemolysis due to deficiency of erythrocyte phosphate dehydrogenase in the newborn. Tetracyclines are contraindicated during pregnancy because of dental staining in the fetus. Thus, the drugs of choice for treatment of UTI in pregnancy are ampicillin and the cephalosporins.

168. The answer is b. (*Rodeck, pp 807–812.*) ATP is an immunologic disorder wherein antibodies to a person's own platelets lead to peripheral destruction of these cells by the reticuloendothelial system, thus leading to reduced numbers of circulating platelets. Platelets continue to be produced in greater-than-normal numbers, leading to large numbers of active young platelets in the circulation that may function to keep the bleeding time close to normal. Because maternal IgG antibody may cross the placenta, coating fetal platelets and leading to thrombocytopenia in the fetus, an atraumatic delivery should be accomplished to protect the fetus. Unfortunately, even cesarean section may not offer complete protection, as at least one case of neonatal hemorrhage and death following cesarean section has been reported. Maternal platelet counts above 100,000 do not guarantee adequate fetal counts.

169. The answer is e. (*Rodeck, pp 865–873.*) Polyhydramnios is an excessive quantity of amniotic fluid. The frequency of diagnosis varies, but polyhydramnios sufficient to cause clinical symptoms probably occurs once in 1000 pregnancies, exclusive of twins. The incidence of associated malformations is about 20% with CNS and GI abnormalities being particularly common. For example, polyhydramnios accompanies about half of cases of anencephaly and nearly all cases of esophageal atresia. Edema of the lower extremities, vulva, and abdominal wall results from compression of major venous systems. Acute hydramnios tends to occur early in pregnancy and, as a rule, leads to labor before the 28th wk. The most frequent maternal complications are placental abruption, uterine dysfunction, and postpartum hemorrhage.

170. The answer is a. (*Gleicher, 3/e, pp 479–488.*) The incidence of acquired immune deficiency syndrome (AIDS) is increasing rapidly in the United States, and AIDS will shortly be among the leading causes of death in women of childbearing age. Since it is associated with multiple sexual partners, other sexually transmitted diseases such as herpes and gonorrhea are relatively common in association with AIDS. Patients with clinical AIDS are at risk for opportunistic infections, the most common of which is *Pneumocystis carinii* pneumonia. Females tend to have a lower median survival than males for the same level of progression of AIDS. Breast feeding is contraindicated because it may be a source of viral transmission to the baby and because maternally derived antibodies can delay diagnosis in the newborn.

171. The answer is e. (*Gleicher, 3/e, pp 1395–1396.*) Worldwide, the incidence of pregnancy-induced hypertension (PIH) varies from a low of 2% in the Far East to almost 30% in Puerto Rico. Peak incidences occur in two groups: young primiparous women and multiparous women who are older than 35 years of age. Moreover, women who have had hypertension of pregnancy in the past have a 33% chance of developing the disease again in later pregnancies. Because of the difficulty in defining normal blood pressure for pregnant women, elevations of 20 mm Hg or more in the systolic component or of 10 mm Hg or more in the diastolic component during pregnancy are defined as abnormal, notwithstanding the absolute blood pressure values. The risk of PIH in subsequent pregnancies is higher when there is a different father, which points toward an immunologic etiology. The terminology regarding hypertension in pregnancy is still in flux; the most inclusive term, hypertensive states of pregnancy, is recommended by the American College of Obstetricians and Gynecologists Committee on Terminology for general use. If the hypertension was not present before conception, then the term *pregnancy-induced hypertension* is also acceptable, but the term *toxemia* has fallen into disfavor.

172. The answer is e. (*Rodeck, pp 112–114.*) Although during early pregnancy the diabetogenic effects of placental hormones are not marked, there is still a net transfer of glucose from mother to fetus. For this reason, there is a tendency toward maternal hypoglycemia rather than hyperglycemia; ketoacidosis is rare and insulin reactions are common. In fact, one of the first symptoms of pregnancy in a diabetic woman may be hypoglycemia and decreasing insulin need. Later on in pregnancy, however, insulin requirements increase markedly and are about two-thirds higher than before pregnancy. Hypoglycemia then becomes less of a problem than ketoacidosis.

173. The answer is c. (*Reece, 2/e, pp 1055–1084.*) Maternal diabetes mellitus can affect a pregnant woman and her fetus in many ways. The development of preeclampsia or eclampsia is about 4 times as likely as among nondiabetic women. Infection is also more likely not only to occur but to be severe. The incidences of fetal macrosomia or death and of dystocia are increased, and hydramnios is common. The likelihood of postpartum hemorrhage after vaginal delivery and the frequency of cesarean section both are increased in diabetic women. The incidence of fetal genetic disorders such as cystic fibrosis is unaffected by diabetes.

174. The answer is c. *(Reece, 2/e, pp 1171–1173.)* Systemic lupus erythematosus (SLE) is a relatively common connective tissue disorder with a prevalence of 1:700 in white women and 1:260 in black women. There is a significant female predominance, with a female-to-male ratio of 10:1. In general, the condition of the patient with SLE is likely to worsen during pregnancy. However, two-thirds of patients who were in remission at least 6 mo before gestation will remain in clinical remission throughout pregnancy. Increased fetal wastage is observed in pregnant women with SLE, most affecting female offspring. Clinical congenital lupus syndromes also occur predominantly in female infants, which suggests that maternally transmitted antibodies may be more toxic to female offspring. Two specific clinical syndromes have been described in pregnant patients with lupus: thrombocytopenia and a preeclampsia-like syndrome with hypertension and proteinuria.

175. The answer is e. *(Reece, 2/e, pp 1055–1084.)* Sophisticated management of high-risk diabetic persons has reduced the incidence of diabetic ketoacidosis. When it occurs in pregnant women, however, it is associated with an extremely high fetal mortality. In addition, ketonuria in the absence of acidosis (i.e., starvation ketosis) has been correlated with decreased intelligence quotients in the offspring. Perinatal mortality has been correlated with hyperglycemia and glycosuria even in the absence of ketoacidosis, and this finding is the cornerstone of current recommendations urging strict control of diabetes during pregnancy. A correlation between maternal hypoglycemia and fetal morbidity or mortality has not been shown; in fact, rather severe episodes of hypoglycemia have been reported to have no effect on the outcome of pregnancy.

176. The answer is c. *(James, 2/e, 805–808.)* Epilepsy affects between 0.3% and 0.6% of pregnant women. In one large series of studies, seizure frequency increased in 45% of patients during pregnancy, was reduced in 5%, and remained unchanged in the rest of the patients. When seizure frequency increased, it most commonly did so during the first trimester. In general, control of patients with frequent seizures before pregnancy was more likely to deteriorate during gestation, but the course in the individual case could not be predicted accurately. Women with epilepsy have a significant risk of stillbirths and fetal malformations, either from the effects of seizure activity (e.g., hypoxia) or from teratogenic effects of anticonvulsive medications. Antiepileptic drugs, such as phenytoin, taken by the mother are usually secreted in breast milk, but their concentration is probably insufficient to have a demonstrable effect on the baby. Thus, breast feeding should not be discouraged in epileptic mothers. However, in early pregnancy, fetuses have a higher risk of anomaly, which must be balanced against an usually greater risk of seizures and fetal harm that may stem from not taking antiepileptic drugs.

177. The answer is d. (*Reece, 2/e, pp 1112.*) Hyperthyroidism in pregnancy may cause neonatal thyrotoxicosis. The mechanism is not the transmission of triiodothyronine or thyroxine to the baby, but rather the crossing of long-acting thyroid stimulator (LATS) to the baby with subsequent hyperfunction of the fetal thyroid gland. Not all hyperthyroid women have LATS; only those who do are at risk for neonatal thyrotoxicosis. The usual treatment for hyperthyroidism in pregnancy is administration of thiourea compounds, although in some centers surgery is popular. Hyperthyroidism often becomes less severe during pregnancy, especially during the last trimester, at which time requirements for thiourea drugs often decrease. Because hyperthyroidism is a treatable disorder, it is not an indication for terminating a pregnancy.

178. The answer is d. (*Reece, 2/3, pp 875–876.*) It is not known why hypothyroidism is uncommon during pregnancy; however, the most widely supported explanation is that many hypothyroid patients are anovulatory, and thus do not easily become pregnant. However, if a hypothyroid patient does become pregnant, her disease, if untreated, could lead to abortion and stillbirth. For this reason, most perinatologists prefer to treat hypothyroidism vigorously during pregnancy. For example, if a woman who has been placed on low-dose thyroid replacement for poorly documented hypothyroidism becomes pregnant, administration of thyroid hormone probably should be increased to full replacement dosage for the remainder of the pregnancy; after delivery, hormone therapy should be discontinued in order to reevaluate thyroid function. Fetal hypothyroidism comes from maternal hypothyroidism.

179. The answer is d. (*James, 2/e, pp 343–359.*) Erythroblastosis fetalis, also known as isoimmune hemolytic disease of the newborn, results from the transplacental passage of maternal blood group antibodies and subsequent destructive reaction with fetal erythrocyte antigens. It is theoretically possible for any blood group antigen, with the exception of Lewis and I antigens, to cause erythroblastosis fetalis. Lewis and I antigens are not present on fetal red blood cells; furthermore, the antibody to these two antigens is immunoglobulin M, which does not cross the placenta.

180. The answer is b. (*Cunningham, 20/e, pp 866, 877–879. Lambrou, pp 58, 17.*) In the twin-twin transfusion syndrome, the donor twin is always anemic, owing not to a hemolytic process but to the direct transfer of blood to the recipient twin, who becomes polycythemic. The recipient may suffer thromboses secondary to hypertransfusion and subsequent hemoconcentration. Although the donor placenta is usually pale and somewhat atrophied, that of the recipient is congested and enlarged. Hydramnios can develop in either twin but, because of circulatory overload, is more frequent in the recipient. When hydramnios occurs in the donor, it is due to congestive heart failure caused by severe anemia.

181. The answer is d. (*Reece, 2/e, p 924–925.*) When an incompetent cervix is suspected, weekly cervical examinations beginning at 16 to 18 wk gestation can reveal evidence of cervical dilatation or effacement in time to perform corrective surgery. The most commonly used techniques are the Shirodkar cervical suture (cerclage), in which the purse-string suture is buried under the vaginal mucosa and the bladder is pushed back for higher placement of the stitch, and the McDonald cervical suture, a simple purse-string suture most widely used when the cervix is well effaced. Once the diagnosis has been made, a cerclage procedure may be performed prophylactically in subsequent pregnancies prior to any change in the cervix. This is best done at 14 to 16 wk, well past the time when spontaneous abortion is common. Because it is not until 16 to 18 wk that the fetus begins to occupy the lower uterine segment, it would be unlikely that an incompetent cervix would be the cause of recurrent pregnancy loss at 14 to 16 wk. Legal abortions are only very rarely related to subsequent cervical incompetence.

182. The answer is e. (*Gleicher, 3/e, pp 27–31.*) Numerous changes occur in the cardiovascular system during pregnancy. Heart rate increases about 10 to 15 beats/min. Blood volume and cardiac output increase significantly. Many cardiac sounds that would be abnormal in a nonpregnant state are normal during pregnancy. All the findings listed in the question are normal.

Ninety percent of pregnant women have systolic ejection murmurs. In approximately 20% of women, a soft diastolic murmur can be heard.

183. The answer is d. *(Queenan, 4/e, pp 79–82.)* Eisenmenger syndrome consists of severe pulmonary hypertension combined with a bidirectional or reversed shunt through a patent ductus arteriosus or an atrial or ventricular septal defect. The death rate during pregnancy for women who have this syndrome is higher than in any other form of congenital heart disease. Death usually occurs at or just after delivery and is probably associated with a sudden drop in peripheral vascular resistance. Atrial and ventricular septal defects, in the absence of pulmonary hypertension and right-to-left shunting, rarely cause problems during pregnancy. Unless shunting is minimal, a patent ductus arteriosus is usually detected by the time a woman becomes pregnant. Again, only reversal of the shunt should pose problems. Wolff-Parkinson-White arrhythmias are usually not incompatible with successful pregnancy.

184. The answer is a. *(Gleicher, 3/e, pp 235–240.)* The development of techniques for multifetal pregnancy reduction has markedly improved the outcome in multifetal pregnancies. The procedure usually is done in the first trimester. After 13 to 14 wk, morbidity and mortality seem to increase substantially. Increased rates of fetal loss and prematurity are associated with higher starting and finishing numbers. The procedure has become safer with increasing operator experience. The technique by which ovulation was induced seems irrelevant.

185. The answer is c. *(James, 2/e, pp 547–548, 623.)* Rifampin has occasionally been known to cause a flulike syndrome, abdominal pain, acute renal failure, and thrombocytopenia. It may also resemble hepatitis and can cause orange urine, sweat, and tears. INH has been associated with hepatitis, hypersensitivity reactions, and peripheral neuropathies. The neuropathy can be prevented by the administration of pyridoxine, especially in the pregnant patient, where pyridoxine requirements are increased. INH may also cause a rash, a fever, and a lupuslike syndrome with a positive ANA titer. Streptomycin has a potential for ototoxicity in both the mother and the fetus. The most commonly seen fetal side effects include minor vestibular impairment, auditory impairment, or both. Cases of severe and bilateral hearing loss and marked vestibular abnormalities have been reported with streptomycin use. Optic neuritis is a well-described side effect of ethambutol, although it is rare at the usual prescribed doses.

186. The answer is e. *(Cunningham, 20/e, pp 701–704, 714.)* Aspirin has been associated with platelet dysfunction and prolonged clotting times in both pregnant and nonpregnant women. Neonatal jaundice secondary to aspirin ingestion is caused by displacement of bilirubin from protein binding sites. The use of analgesic compounds that contain aspirin has also been associated with postdated gestations, but does not affect amniotic fluid volume.

187. The answer is b. *(Hankins, pp 576–584.)* The treatment of the apparently incompetent cervix is surgical, and consists of reinforcing the weak cervix by some kind of purse-string suture. It is best performed after the first trimester, but before cervical dilatation of 4 cm, if possible. Bleeding, infection, and uterine contractions are contraindications to surgery.

ANTEPARTUM SURVEILLANCE, LABOR, AND DELIVERY

Questions

DIRECTIONS: Each item below contains a question or incomplete statement followed by suggested responses. Select the **one best** response to each question.

188. The smallest anteroposterior diameter of the pelvic inlet is called the

a. Interspinous diameter
b. True conjugate
c. Diagonal conjugate
d. Obstetric conjugate

189. A pelvis that is characterized by an anteroposterior diameter of the inlet greater than the transverse diameter is classified as

a. Gynecoid
b. Android
c. Anthropoid
d. Platypelloid

190. An abnormal attitude is illustrated by

a. Breech presentation
b. Face presentation
c. Transverse position
d. Occiput posterior
e. Occiput anterior

191. In which of the following fetal presentations can a vaginal delivery occur at term?

a. Face presentation with the chin immediately under the symphysis pubis
b. Face presentation with the chin rotated directly posteriorly
c. Brow presentation
d. Shoulder presentation

192. The frequency of breech presentation at term is

a. 1% to 2%
b. 3% to 4%
c. 5% to 6%
d. 7% to 8%
e. 9% to 10%

193. Which of the following statements regarding management of labor in a low-risk pregnancy is true?

a. Amniotomy may shorten the length of labor slightly, but not as much as spontaneous rupture
b. Universal electronic fetal monitoring improves perinatal outcome
c. Food and oral fluids are acceptable if labor is progressing normally
d. An indwelling catheter is frequently needed when the patient is unable to void spontaneously

194. Which of the following statements regarding monitoring of fetal heart rate (FHR) is true?

a. A sinusoidal FHR pattern is almost invariably associated with an anemic, asphyxiated fetus
b. A saltatory FHR pattern is almost invariably seen during rather than before labor
c. The FHR tracing of the premature fetus should be analyzed by different criteria than tracings obtained at term
d. Fetuses with congenital anomalies will invariably exhibit abnormal FHR patterns

195. Hypertonic dysfunctional labor generally can be expected to

a. Be associated with rapid cervical dilation
b. Cause little pain
c. Occur in the active phase of labor
d. React favorably to oxytocin stimulation
e. Respond to sedation

196. Acute obstruction of the umbilical circulation has been found experimentally to result in which of the following responses?

a. A rapid fall in fetal central venous pressure
b. Short-term maintenance of fetal heart rate
c. A rapidly mediated humoral effect on the fetal heart
d. A rapidly mediated response by the fetal heart that can be affected by cutting the vagi
e. Systolic/diastolic (S/D) changes secondary to a fall in central venous pressure

197. Which of the following influences the incidence of fetal breathing movement in the third trimester in the IUGR fetus, but not an advanced-gestational-age fetus?

a. Maternal hypercapnia
b. Maternal glucose concentration
c. Time of day at which measurements are made
d. Maternal hyperoxia

198. Following a cesarean birth, contraindications for a trial of labor in a subsequent pregnancy include

a. Breech presentation
b. Lack of a prior vaginal delivery
c. The fact that the first section was for cephalopelvic disproportion (CPD)
d. Unavailability of x-ray pelvimetry
e. Classic cesarean section scar

199. A forceps rotation of 30° from left occiput anterior (OA) to OA with extraction of the fetus from +2 station would be described as which type of delivery?

a. Outlet forceps
b. Low forceps
c. Midforceps
d. High forceps

DIRECTIONS: Each group of questions below consists of lettered options followed by numbered items. For each numbered item, select the appropriate lettered option(s). Each lettered option may be used once, more than once, or not at all. **Choose exactly the number of options indicated following each item.**

Items 200–202

For each clinical situation that follows, select the most likely placental disorder.

a. Placenta accreta
b. Placenta circumvallata
c. Placenta membranacea
d. Placenta succenturiata
e. Vasa previa

200. A 24-year-old woman, gravida 2, para 1, goes into premature labor at 33 wk gestation after an apparently normal antepartum course **(SELECT 1 DISORDER)**

201. An apparently normal pregnancy culminates in the spontaneous delivery of an infant who weighs 3.2 kg (7 lb) with Apgars of 9/9. The placenta delivers spontaneously followed by an unusual amount of uterine bleeding. **(SELECT 1 DISORDER)**

202. After the low forceps delivery of an infant who weighs 1.8 kg (4 lb) to a 27-year-old woman, gravida 4, para 3 (whose second baby was born by cesarean section owing to fetal distress but whose third baby delivered vaginally), the placenta does not deliver spontaneously. After 20 min the obstetrician attempts a manual removal but is unable to identify a plane of cleavage. **(SELECT 1 DISORDER)**

Items 203–205

For each clinical situation described, choose the appropriate type of breech position.

a. Complete breech
b. Incomplete breech
c. Frank breech
d. Single footling breech
e. Double footling breech

203. Lower extremities are flexed at the hips and extended at the knees with the feet lying close to the fetal head **(SELECT 1 POSITION)**

204. Lower extremities are flexed at the hips, and one or both knees are flexed **(SELECT 1 POSITION)**

205. The most common breech presentation near term **(SELECT 1 POSITION)**

206. Which of the following abnormalities of labor is associated with a significantly increased incidence of neonatal morbidity?

a. Prolonged latent phase
b. Protracted descent
c. Secondary arrest of dilation
d. Protracted active-phase dilation

207. The one measurement of maturity that is not effected by a "bloody tap" at the time of amniocentesis is

a. Lecithin-to-sphingomyelin (L/S) ratio
b. α fetoprotein
c. Bilirubin as measured by DOD_{450}
d. Phosphatidyl glycerol

208. In the evaluation of a fetus with intrauterine growth retardation, Doppler ultrasound of which of the following vessels is likely to suggest impending fetal distress?

a. Circle of Willis
b. Middle cerebral artery
c. Carotid artery
d. Internal placental vessels
e. Renal artery

209. Fetal pulmonary maturity can be evaluated by phospholipid activity in amniotic fluid. In which of the following pregnancies does the fetus have the *least* chance of developing respiratory distress syndrome (RDS)?

a. Normal pregnancy; amniotic fluid L/S is 1.8:1, phosphatidyl glycerol (PG) is absent
b. Hypertensive pregnancy; amniotic fluid L/S is 1.8:1, PG is absent
c. Hypertensive pregnancy; amniotic fluid L/S is 2:1, PG is absent
d. Diabetic pregnancy; amniotic fluid L/S is 2:1, PG is present

210. Doppler studies of the umbilical circulation

a. Show that changes in flow velocity waveforms of the umbilical artery may be important in clinical management of high-risk pregnancies
b. Exhibit in normal pregnancy a characteristic increase in the systolic/diastolic (S/D) ratio with advancing gestational age
c. Report a decrease in S/D ratio resulting from nicotine and maternal smoking
d. Show that absence of end-diastolic flow is normal at term
e. Do not have a place in the clinical management of multiple gestations

211. The most likely correlate of hypoxic ischemic encephalopathy attributable to hypoxia at the time of birth is

a. Cerebral palsy
b. Neonatal neurologic sequelae such as hypertonia
c. An Apgar score of less than 3 at 1 min
d. Multiple organ system dysfunction
e. Respiratory acidemia with pH less than 7.2

212. Which of the following does not cause elevated resting pressures?

a. Placental abruption
b. Placenta previa
c. Cephalopelvic disproportion
d. Oxytocin (Pitocin) hyperstimulation
e. Fetal malpresentation

Items 213–217

Match each description with the appropriate fetal heart rate tracing. If none of the tracings apply, answer e (none).

213. Hyperstimulation **(SELECT 1 TRACING)**

214. Early deceleration **(SELECT 1 TRACING)**

215. Acceleration with normal variability **(SELECT 1 TRACING)**

216. Variable deceleration with late component **(SELECT 1 TRACING)**

217. Late deceleration with flat baseline (**SELECT 1 TRACING**)

a.

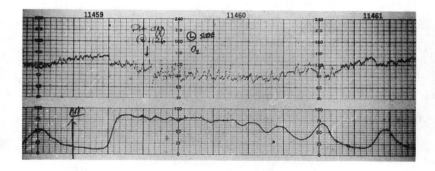

b.

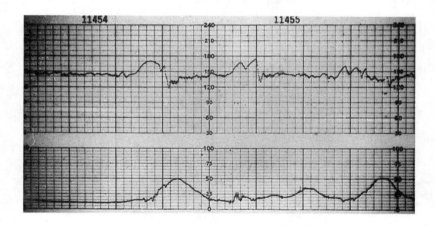

c.

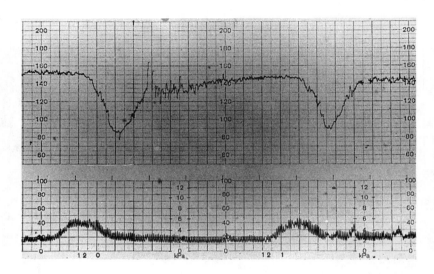

d.

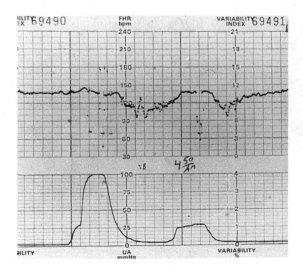

218. Which of the following statements concerning the use of magnesium sulfate in pregnancy is true?

a. Magnesium sulfate is an effective antihypertensive agent when used at serum levels to prevent convulsions
b. A therapeutic range of 7 to 10 meq/L is necessary to prevent convulsions
c. An intramuscular regimen of magnesium sulfate can result in therapeutic levels as effectively as continuous IV infusion
d. Magnesium will not enter the fetal circulation
e. Monitoring the presence of the patellar reflex is a poor indicator of magnesium sulfate levels

219. Which of the following is most likely to be associated with aspiration pneumonitis

a. Fasting during labor
b. Antacid medications prior to anesthesia
c. Endotracheal intubation
d. Extubation with the patient in the lateral recumbent position with her head lowered
e. Extubation with the patient in the semierect position (semi-Fowler's)

220. Which of the following is the most appropriate management of a face presentation with no fetal distress and an adequate pelvis, as determined by digital examination?

a. Perform immediate cesarean section without labor
b. Allow spontaneous labor with vaginal delivery
c. Perform forceps rotation in the second stage of labor to convert mentum posterior to mentum anterior and to allow vaginal delivery
d. Allow to labor spontaneously until complete cervical dilatation is achieved and then perform an internal podalic version with breech extraction
e. Attempt manual conversion of the face to vertex in the second stage of labor

221. A 24-year-old G1, P0, Rh-negative patient is at 36 wk with a breech presentation and is considering external cephalic version. She should be told that

a. She should be offered general anesthesia
b. The procedure can be done with oligohydramnios
c. Prophylaxis with antiglobulin D can wait until after delivery
d. Engagement of the presenting part is not considered a contraindication to version
e. Tocolysis with intravenous ritodrine has been shown to improve the results of external version

Items 222–223

The graph below portrays a labor curve for a woman, gravida 3, para 2, at 39 wk gestation. Membranes were ruptured at 4 cm. The fluid was clear and there has been no indication of fetal distress. Previous infants weighed 3500 g and 3750 g. The estimated weight of this infant, which appears normal on ultrasound, is 3200 g.

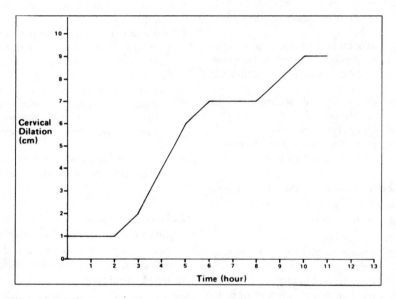

222. This labor curve is compatible with which of the following conditions?

a. Prolonged latent phase
b. Protracted active phase dilation
c. Hypertonic dysfunction
d. Secondary arrest of dilation
e. Primary dysfunction

223. In the clinical situation described above, an intrauterine pressure catheter shows a contraction frequency of 2 per 10 min with an amplitude of 35 mm Hg. The preferred management is

a. Ambulation
b. Sedation
c. Administration of oxytocin
d. Cesarean section
e. Expectant

224. A primipara is in labor and an episiotomy is about to be cut. Compared with a midline episiotomy, an advantage of mediolateral episiotomy is

a. Ease of repair
b. Fewer breakdowns
c. Lower blood loss
d. Less dyspareunia
e. Less extension of the incision

225. A 17-year-old primipara at 41 wk wants an immediate cesarean section. She is also being followed with biophysical profile testing. You tell her that

a. It includes amniotic fluid volume, fetal breathing, fetal body movements, fetal body tone, and contraction stress testing
b. The false negative rate of the biophysical profile is 10%
c. False positive results on biophysical profile are rare
d. Spontaneous decelerations during biophysical profile testing are associated with significant fetal morbidity
e. A normal biophysical profile should be repeated in 1 wk to 10 days in a postterm pregnancy

226. Advantages of a lower-segment vertical uterine incision over a lower-segment transverse incision include which of the following?

a. Less blood loss
b. Ease of repair
c. Less likelihood of adhesion to bowel or omentum along the incision line
d. Less likelihood of dehiscence
e. Less likelihood of tearing into the uterine artery

227. A 27-year-old woman (gravida 3, para 2) comes to the delivery floor at 37 wk gestation. She has had no prenatal care. She complains that, on bending down to pick up her 2-year-old child, she experienced sudden, severe back pain. This pain now has persisted for 2 h. Approximately 30 min ago she noted bright red blood coming from her vagina. By the time she arrives at the delivery floor, she is contracting strongly every 3 min; the uterus is quite firm even between contractions. By abdominal palpation the fetus is vertex with the head deeply engaged. Fetal heart rate is 130 beats/min. The fundus is 38 cm above the symphysis. Blood for clotting is drawn, and a clot forms in 4 min. Clotting studies are sent to the laboratory. Which of the following actions can wait until the patient is stabilized?

a. Stabilizing maternal circulation
b. Attaching a fetal electronic monitor
c. Inserting an intrauterine pressure catheter
d. Administering heparin immediately
e. Preparing for cesarean section

Items 228–230

For each of the following clinical descriptions, select the procedure that is most appropriate.

a. External version
b. Internal version
c. Midforceps rotation
d. Low transverse cesarean section
e. Classic cesarean section

228. A 24-year-old primigravid woman, at term, has been in labor for 16 h and has been dilated to 9 cm for 3 h. The fetal vertex is in the right occiput posterior position, at +1 station, and molded. There have been mild late decelerations for the last 30 min. Twenty minutes ago the fetal scalp pH was 7.27; it is now 7.20. **(SELECT 1 PROCEDURE)**

229. You have just delivered an infant weighing 2.5 kg (5.5 lb) at 39 wk gestation. Because the uterus still feels large, you do a vaginal examination. A second set of membranes is bulging through a fully dilated cervix, and you feel a small part presenting in the sac. A fetal heart is auscultated at 60 beats/min. **(SELECT 1 PROCEDURE)**

230. A 24-year-old woman (gravida 3, para 2) is at 40 wk gestation. The fetus is in the transverse lie presentation. **(SELECT 1 PROCEDURE)**

Items 231–233

Choose the appropriate treatment for each clinical situation described below.

a. Epidural block
b. Meperidine (Demerol), 100 mg intramuscularly
c. Oxytocin intravenously
d. Midforceps delivery
e. Cesarean section

231. A multiparous woman has had painful uterine contractions every 2 to 4 min for the last 17 h. The cervix is dilated to 2 to 3 cm and effaced 50%; it has not changed since admission. (**SELECT 1 TREATMENT**)

232. A nulliparous woman is in active labor (cervical dilatation 5 cm with complete effacement, the vertex at 0 station); the labor curve shows protracted progression without descent following the administration of an epidural block. An intrauterine pressure catheter shows contractions every 4 to 5 min, peaking at 40 mm Hg. (**SELECT 1 TREATMENT**)

233. A 59-10 nulliparous woman has had arrest of descent for the last 2 h and arrest of dilation for the last 3 h. The cervix is dilated to 7 cm and the vertex is at 21 station. Monitoring shows a normal pattern and adequate contractions. Fetal weight is estimated at 7.5 lb. (**SELECT 1 TREATMENT**)

Items 234–237

Match each description with the most appropriate type of obstetric anesthesia.

a. Paracervical block
b. Pudendal block
c. Spinal block
d. Epidural block

234. Appears to lengthen the second stage of labor (**SELECT 1 BLOCK**)

235. Is frequently associated with fetal bradycardia (**SELECT 1 BLOCK**)

236. May be complicated by profound hypotension (**SELECT 1 BLOCK**)

237. May be associated with increased need for augmentation of labor with oxytocin and for instrument-assisted delivery (**SELECT 1 BLOCK**)

ANTEPARTUM SURVEILLANCE, LABOR, AND DELIVERY

Answers

188. The answer is d. (*Cunningham, 20/e, pp 60–62.*) The obstetric conjugate is the shortest distance between the promontory of the sacrum and the symphysis pubis. It generally measures 10.5 cm. Because the obstetric conjugate cannot be clinically measured, it is estimated by subtracting 1.5 to 2.0 cm from the diagonal conjugate, which is the distance from the lower margin of the symphysis to the sacral promontory. The true conjugate is measured from the top of the symphysis to the sacral promontory. The interspinous diameter is the transverse measurement of the midplane and generally is the smallest diameter of the pelvis.

189. The answer is c. (*Cunningham, 20/e, pp 60–62.*) By tradition, pelves are classified as belonging to one of four major groups. The gynecoid pelvis is the classic female pelvis with a posterior sagittal diameter of the inlet only slightly shorter than the anterior sagittal. In the android pelvis, the posterior sagittal diameter at the inlet is much shorter than the anterior sagittal, limiting the use of the posterior space by the fetal head. In the anthropoid pelvis the anteroposterior (AP) diameter of the inlet is greater than the transverse, resulting in an oval with large sacrosciatic notches and convergent side walls. Ischial spines are likely to be prominent. The platypelloid pelvis is flattened with a short AP and wide transverse diameter. Wide sacrosciatic notches are common. The pelves of most women do not fall into a pure type and are blends of one or more of the above types.

190. The answer is b. (*Cunningham, 20/e, pp 253–254.*) Lie of the fetus refers to the relation of the long axis of the fetus to that of the mother and is classified as longitudinal, transverse, or oblique. The fetal attitude refers to the fetal posture—either flexed or extended. A face presentation results from an extension of the fetus's neck. Presentation refers to the portion of the baby that is foremost in the birth canal. Occiput transverse and occiput anterior are examples of positions—that is, relative relationships of the fetus to the mother.

191. The answer is a. *(Cunningham, 20/e, pp 253–255.)* In a face presentation, the object of internal rotation is to bring the chin under the symphysis pubis. Unless the head is unusually small, natural delivery cannot otherwise be accomplished. Only in this way can the neck subtend the posterior surface of the symphysis pubis. If the chin rotates directly posteriorly, the relatively short neck cannot span the anterior surface of the sacrum. Birth of the head is impossible unless the fetus is markedly premature or macerated. A brow presentation occupies a position midway between full flexion and full extension. Unless the fetus is small or the pelvis unusually large, engagement of the head and subsequent delivery cannot take place as long as this presentation persists. A shoulder presentation occurs with a transverse lie. The spontaneous birth of a fully developed infant is impossible in this position.

192. The answer is b. *(Cunningham, 20/e, pp 251, 496.)* At term, approximately 96% of fetuses are in vertex presentation. About two-thirds of all vertex presentations are in the left occiput position. About 3% to 4% of fetuses at term are in breech presentation. Face and shoulder presentations constitute 0.3% and 0.4%, respectively.

193. The answer is a. *(Reece, 2/e, p 1630.)* Amniotomy may shorten the labor slightly, but not as much as spontaneous rupture of membranes. There is no evidence whatsoever that shorter labor is beneficial to mother or fetus. Universal use of electronic fetal monitoring has not been found to reduce the incidence of perinatal asphyxia, low Apgar scores, or perinatal death. When a group of patients with universal fetal monitoring in labor was compared with one in which electronic fetal monitoring was applied only to selected cases, the only documented difference was in increased incidence of abnormal FHR patterns and cesarean deliveries performed for fetal distress in the former group. Food and oral fluids should be withheld during active labor and delivery since gastric emptying time is prolonged by established labor and analgesics and food remaining in the stomach increases the likelihood of vomiting and aspiration. Bladder distention during labor must be avoided since it can lead to both obstructed labor and bladder hypotonia. If the bladder is palpated during examination, the patient should be encouraged to void. If she cannot, intermittent catheterization may be indicated. The use of an indwelling catheter should be avoided, however, since it increases the risk of urinary tract infection.

194. The answer is b. (*Queenan, 4/e, pp 177–179.*) The sinusoidal pattern was first described in a group of severely affected Rh-isoimmunized fetuses. It has also been described, however, in normal fetuses and in association with maternal medication (e.g., alphaprodine). A saltatory pattern, which in the past was associated with depressed fetuses with low Apgar scores, is now thought to represent episodes of brief and acute hypoxia in the previously normally oxygenated fetus. This pattern is almost invariably seen during rather than before labor. The same relationship between the FHR pattern and the acid-base status has been documented in preterm and in term fetuses. Thus, both the antepartum and the intrapartum FHR patterns of the premature fetus should be analyzed by the same criteria used at term. The vast majority of fetuses with congenital anomalies have normal FHR patterns and a response to asphyxia similar to that of the normal fetus. Although no pathognomonic abnormal FHR patterns have been described for such fetuses, the rate of cesarean sections for fetal distress is reported to be significantly increased in this group. This may be explained by the oligohydramnios and fetal growth retardation that commonly occur in pregnancies affected by fetal congenital anomalies.

195. The answer is e. (*Cunningham, 20/e, pp 421–422.*) Hypertonic uterine dysfunction is characterized by a lack of coordination of uterine contractions, possibly caused by disorganization of the contraction gradient, which normally is greatest at the fundus and least at the cervix. This type of dysfunction usually appears during the latent phase of labor and is responsive to sedation, not oxytocin stimulation. The disorder is accompanied by a great deal of discomfort with little cervical dilation (the familiar and painful false labor). After being sedated for a few hours, affected women usually awaken in active labor.

196. The answer is d. (*Reece, 2/e, pp 813–815.*) Fetal heart rate has been shown to drop almost immediately when the umbilical circulation has been obstructed in experimental situations. This response is a reflex action that is caused by the sudden rise in central venous pressure and that disappears if the vagi are severed. A more prolonged obstruction of the umbilical circulation can cause a delayed fall in the fetal heart rate secondary to progressive asphyxia, which will affect the S/D rates.

197. The answer is d. (*Cunningham, 20/e, pp 18, 1011–1018.*) Breathing movements in the human fetus are episodic and occur about 30% of the time in the third trimester. Fetal breathing activity is increased by maternal carbohydrate intake or intravenous glucose load. In the third trimester, the incidence of fetal breathing activity is significantly altered by the time of day at which measurements are made. The percentage of time a fetus spends breathing is increased significantly 2 to 3 h following the mother's meals. This change in breathing patterns appears to follow the normal postprandial increase in maternal blood glucose concentration. Maternal hypercapnia also increases the frequency of fetal breathing movements at term, probably as a result of maturation of fetal respiratory centers. This response is not always present in the fetus that is small for gestational age or premature. In normal fetuses, increasing maternal P_{0_2} does not appear to affect fetal respiratory activity. In contrast, the growth-retarded fetus may respond to maternal hyperoxia with an increase in fetal breathing activity.

198. The answer is e. (*Hankins, pp 305–307.*) Guidelines from the American College of Obstetricians and Gynecologists state that a patient with a prior low transverse cesarean section may attempt a vaginal delivery following informed consent to the risks involved. Although the issue of prior cesarean section for CPD is controversial, this prior procedure is not an absolute contraindication for a trial of labor. A classic incision is a contraindication because of a high risk of uterine rupture. X-ray pelvimetry is not required prior to a trial of labor; a prior vaginal delivery is not necessary either.

199. The answer is b. (*Hankins, pp 129–130, 137–138.*) In the late 1980s and early 1990s, the classic definitions of forceps deliveries were slightly altered to conform with obstetric reality and the need for realistic definitions of procedures vis-à-vis both medical and legal guidelines and standards. Outlet forceps delivery requires a visible scalp, the fetal skull on the pelvic floor, the sagittal suture in essentially OA position, and the fetal head on the perineum. A rotation can occur, but only up to 45°. A low forceps delivery requires a station of at least +2 but not on the pelvic floor. Rotation can be more than 45°. Midforceps delivery is from a station above +2, but with an engaged head. High forceps delivery, for which there are no modern indications, would reflect a head not engaged.

200–202. The answers are 200-b, 201-d, 202-a. *(Cunningham, 20/e, pp 669–670.)* A circumvallate placenta contains a grayish-white ring located a variable distance from the edge of the placenta. The membranes (amnion and chorion) are folded over at this ring and are not in contact with the substance of the placenta peripheral to the ring. The fetal vessels do not go beyond the ring. Placenta circumvallata is associated with an increased rate of prematurity; why the rate is increased is unknown. A succenturiate placenta is characterized by an accessory lobe apart from the main body of the placenta. Fetal vessels usually course through the membranes between the main and accessory lobes and can be identified on inspection of the membranes. If the fetal vessels on their way between the lobes should pass over the cervix, vasa previa occurs. This condition is potentially dangerous because the membranes may rupture, in turn rupturing a fetal vessel and causing fetal hemorrhage. If a succenturiate lobe is left within the uterus after the main body of the placenta has been delivered, postpartum hemorrhage can result; therefore, an accessory lobe should be sought by intrauterine exploration. Placenta accreta is a condition in which the usual plane of cleavage (Nitabuch layer) between the placenta and decidua is absent and the villi attach to the myometrium. It is more common in women who have uterine scars, such as in the patient described in the question, and who have undergone previous cesarean section. Complications of placenta accreta are in part iatrogenic. An overly vigorous attempt at manual removal may cause uterine inversion or perforation and severe bleeding. A hysterectomy may be necessary, although leaving the placenta in place and treating the patient with methotrexate may suffice. Severe complications are most common with the more severe forms of placenta accreta. These forms are known as placenta increta if the villi grow into the muscle of the uterus and placenta percreta if the placenta grows through the myometrium.

203–205. The answers are 203-c, 204-a, 205-c. *(Cunningham, 20/e, pp 495–508.)* Correctly diagnosing the type of breech presentation is critical for management of delivery. In the frank breech presentation, the lower extremities are flexed at the hip and extended at the knees with the feet lying near the fetal head. In the complete breech presentation, the fetus has both hips flexed, with one or both knees flexed. In the incomplete breech presentation, one or both hips are flexed and one (single footling) or both (double footling) feet or knees lie below the breech. The frank breech is the most common breech presentation at term. The incidence of cord prolapse is less in the frank breech presentation than other breech presentations. Most obstetricians elect to deliver the incomplete (single or double footling) breech via cesarean section. Vaginal delivery is sometimes performed in the event of frank or incomplete breech presentation after a diligent search for any other complication that may indicate a cesarean delivery.

206. The answer is c. (*Cunningham, 20/e, pp 421–422.*) Three significant advances in the treatment of uterine dysfunction have reduced the risk of perinatal morbidity and mortality: (1) the avoidance of undue prolongation of labor; (2) the use of intravenous oxytocin in the treatment of some patterns of uterine dysfunction; and (3) the liberal use of cesarean section (rather than midforceps) to effect delivery when oxytocin fails. Prolonged latent phase is not associated with increased risk of perinatal morbidity (PNM) or low Apgar scores and should be treated by therapeutic rest. Protraction disorders have a higher rate of PNM and low Apgar scores, but not if spontaneous labor follows the abnormality. Arrest disorders are associated with significantly higher rates of PNM following either spontaneous or instrument-assisted delivery.

207. The answer is d. (*Reece, 2/e, pp 109–111.*) Blood contaminating the amniotic fluid may appreciably complicate several studies and interpretations of the results. Maternal serum has an L/S ratio of 1:3 to 1:5, and its addition to amniotic fluid influences the ratio accordingly. Meconium lowers the L/S ratio somewhat. Phosphatidyl glycerol has not been detected in blood, meconium, or vaginal secretions; consequently these contaminants do not confuse the interpretation. Minute amounts of fetal (but not maternal) blood can lead to falsely high levels of α fetoprotein in amniotic fluid. For DOD_{450}, a small amount of blood will not seriously jeopardize the accuracy of analysis. Larger amounts of blood, particularly if there is so much that the specimen clots, may falsely lower the 450-μ peak.

208. The answer is e. (*Jaffe, pp 183–205.*) In the fetus with retarded growth, a brain-sparing effect can be noted on ultrasound. Intracranial vessels are less sensitive to the sudden changes in resistance and flow that may signal impending fetal distress in peripheral vessels. Intraplacental blood flow is neither well understood nor documentable and is therefore not clinically useful under such circumstances. Doppler flow changes precede fetal heart rate tracings by as much as several weeks. Changes in cerebral blood flow can and do occur, but are less reliable than changes in peripheral vessels.

209. The answer is a. (*Jaffe, pp 14–15, 252–254.*) Simple, continuous-wave Doppler ultrasound can be used to display flow velocity waveforms as a function of time. With increased gestational age, in normal pregnancy there is an increase in end-diastolic flow velocity relative to peak systolic velocity, which causes the S/D ratio to decrease with advancing gestation. An increase in S/D ratio is associated with increased resistance in the placental vascular bed as can be noted in preeclampsia or fetal growth retardation. Nicotine and maternal smoking have also been reported to increase the S/D ratio. Many studies document the value of umbilical Doppler flow studies in recognition of fetal compromise. It seems that the S/D ratio increases as the fetal condition deteriorates; this is most severe in cases of absent or reversed diastolic flow. In normal twins, the S/D ratio falls within the normal range for singletons. Doppler studies have been used for intensive surveillance in cases of twin-to-twin transfusion.

210. The answer is d. (*Reece, 2/e, pp 109–111.*) The lecithin-to-sphingomyelin (L/S) ratio in amniotic fluid is close to 1 until about 34 wk of gestation, when the concentration of lecithin begins to rise. For pregnancies of unknown duration but otherwise uncomplicated, the risk of respiratory distress syndrome (RDS) is relatively minor when the L/S is at least 2:1. Maternal hypertensive disorders and fetal growth retardation may accelerate the rate of fetal pulmonary maturation, possibly as a result of chronic fetal stress. A delay in fetal pulmonary maturation is observed in pregnancies complicated by maternal diabetes or erythroblastosis fetalis. A risk of RDS of 40% exists with an L/S ratio of 1.5 to 2; when the L/S ratio is <1.5, the risk of RDS is 73%. When the L/S ratio is >2, the risk of RDS is slight. However, when the fetus is likely to have a serious metabolic compromise at birth (e.g., diabetes or sepsis), RDS may develop even with a "mature" L/S ratio (>2.0). This may be explained by lack of PG, a phospholipid that enhances surfactant properties. The identification of PG in amniotic fluid provides considerable reassurance (but not an absolute guarantee) that RDS will not develop.

Moreover, contamination of amniotic fluid by blood, meconium, or vaginal secretions will not alter PG measurements.

211. The answer is d. *(Cunningham, 20/e, pp 976–981.)* Despite the continuing association in medical-legal claims of birth asphyxia and cerebral palsy, the overwhelming preponderance of evidence suggests that birth asphyxia is a very small component. Metabolic or mixed acidemia with pH less than 7; persistent Apgar scores of less than 3 for more than 5 min; seizures, coma, or hypertonia in the newborn; and the appearance of multiple organ system dysfunction could suggest a serious recent insult.

212. The answer is b. *(Reece, 2/e, pp 813–815.)* Normal resting intrauterine pressures are listed as less than 5 mm Hg in the latent phase, less than 12 mm Hg in the active phase, and less than 20 mm Hg in the second stage of labor. Placental abruption, cephalopelvic disproportion, oxytocin (Pitocin) hyperstimulation, fetal malpresentation, and other conditions can cause elevated pressures. Placenta previa, except in association with abruption, does not affect intrauterine pressure.

213–217. The answers are 213-a, 214-e, 215-b, 216-c, 217-d. *(Reece, 2/e, pp 813–815.)* Fetal heart rate tracings are obtained in most pregnancies in the United States through the use of electronic fetal monitoring equipment. Accurate interpretation of these tracings with resultant action taken to expedite delivery in fetuses threatened by hypoxemia has certainly improved neonatal outcome, although it has had very little effect on the overall incidence of cerebral palsy, which seems most often to have its etiology remote from the time of labor. Tracing A shows a classic hyperstimulation pattern with a tonic contraction lasting several minutes with distinctly raised intrauterine pressure, and a consequent fall in fetal heart rate. Despite the increased pressure, there remains good beat-to-beat variability, which suggests that the fetus is withstanding the stress. Tracing B shows fetal heart rate accelerations occurring spontaneously both before and after contractions, with good beat-to-beat variability, and is representative of a very healthy fetus. Tracing C shows variable decelerations with a late component in which the classic V-shaped picture of a variable deceleration is maintained, but the first deceleration on the left shows a prolonged recovery of several minutes before actually reaching the original baseline.

Such compound decelerations are not as ominous as classic late decelerations, but bear careful scrutiny. Tracing D shows late decelerations following two consecutive contractions. While the decrement in fetal heart rate is not great, it is seen in both contractions. The baseline variability is significantly reduced, and this is a very ominous pattern.

218. The answer is c. (*Cunningham, 20/e, pp 722–725.*) The appropriate use of MgSO$_4$ · 7H$_2$O will nearly always arrest eclamptic seizures and prevent recurrences. A therapeutic range of 4 to 7 meq/L will prevent convulsions, and it can be achieved adequately and safely by either intravenous or intramuscular routes of administration after a loading dose of 10 g intramuscularly or 4 g intravenously. Maintenance is best achieved with a continuous intravenous infusion of 2 g/h or a 5-g intramuscular injection every 4 h. Monitoring the presence or absence of the patellar reflex, which disappears at 10 meq/L, is an accurate means of determining the magnesium level. Respiratory arrest will occur at levels above 12 meq/L. Magnesium ions will enter the fetal circulation and will equilibrate with maternal plasma levels. Magnesium sulfate in dosages used to prevent convulsions has no significant antihypertensive effect.

219. The answer is e. (*Cunningham, 20/e, p 1108. Dewan, pp 3–5.*) Aspiration pneumonitis is the most common cause of anesthetic-related death in obstetrics. Its occurrence may be minimized by reducing both the volume and acidity of gastric contents, which is often difficult in the patient in labor whose stomach is extremely slow to empty. All obstetric patients should be intubated for general anesthesia by a skilled professional. Extubation must be accomplished only after the patient is fully conscious and recumbent with her head turned to the side and lowered below the level of her chest.

220. The answer is b. (*Cunningham, 20/e, pp 251, 443–445.*) In the event of a face presentation, successful vaginal delivery will occur the majority of the time with an adequate pelvis. Spontaneous internal rotation during labor is required to bring the chin to the anterior position, which allows the neck to pass beneath the pubis. Therefore, the patient is allowed to labor spontaneously; a cesarean section is employed for failure to progress or for fetal distress. Manual conversion to vertex, forceps rotation, and internal version are no longer employed in obstetrics to deliver the face presentation because of undue trauma to both the mother and the fetus.

221. The answer is e. *(Cunningham, 20/e, pp 505–506.)* The use of external cephalic version is gaining popularity as a safe alternative to term breech presentation, and it is recommended by many, but not all, obstetricians in uncomplicated pregnancies with a breech or a transverse lie after 36 wk. The criteria for a safe and successful external version include continuous monitoring of fetal heart rate, a nonirritable uterus, a sufficient quantity of amniotic fluid, and a presenting part that is not engaged in the pelvis. The availability of ultrasound and the capability of performing an emergency cesarean section are also strongly recommended. The use of tocolytics is advocated and has been shown to improve the success of version, especially on repeat versions after a previous failure. General anesthesia is contraindicated because of the likelihood of trauma to the mother and the fetus. Antiglobulin D prophylaxis is recommended prior to external version in all Rh-negative women because of the risk of fetal-maternal bleeding with manipulation of the uterus.

222–223. The answers are 222-d, 223-c. *(Scott, 8/e, pp 438–444.)* The labor portrayed in this labor curve is characteristic of a secondary arrest of dilation. The woman has entered the active phase of labor as she previously progressed from 2 to 6 cm in less than 2 h. The multiparous woman normally progresses at a rate of at least 1.5 cm/h (and the nullipara at least 1.2 cm/h) in the active phase. Dilation at a slower rate is a protraction disorder. Primary dysfunction, prolonged latent phase, and hypertonic dysfunction occur prior to the active phase. The best evidence available indicates that this labor is hypotonic. Since the ultrasound indicates a fetus without obvious abnormalities and since the patient's previous infants were larger than this one, we assume the absence of cephalopelvic disproportion (CPD). Oxytocin is the treatment of choice. If CPD were suspected, then the treatment preferred by many obstetricians would be cesarean section.

224. The answer is e. *(Hankins, pp 106–122.)* Midline episiotomies are easier to fix and have a smaller incidence of surgical breakdown, less pain, and lower blood loss. The incidence of dyspareunia is somewhat less. However, the incidence of extensions of the incision to include the rectum is considerably higher than with mediolateral episiotomies. Regardless of technique, attention to hemostasis and anatomic restoration is the key element of a technically appropriate repair.

225. The answer is d. *(Cunningham, 20/e, pp 1012–1018.)* The biophysical profile is based on FHR monitoring (generally nonstress testing) in addition to four parameters observed on real-time ultrasonography: amniotic fluid volume, fetal breathing, fetal body movements, and fetal body tones. Each parameter gets a score of 0 to 2. A score of 8 to 10 is considered normal, a score of 6 is equivocal, and a score of 4 or less is abnormal and prompts delivery. The false negative rate for the biophysical profile is less than 0.1%, but false positive results are relatively frequent, with poor specificity. Oligohydramnios is an ominous sign, as are spontaneous decelerations. In patients with profile scores of 8 but with spontaneous decelerations, the rate of cesarean delivery indicated for fetal distress has been 25%. Testing more frequently than every 7 days is recommended in patients with postterm pregnancies, connective tissue disease, chronic hypertension, and suspected fetal growth retardation, as well as in patients with previous fetal death.

226. The answer is e. *(Hankins, pp 311–324.)* The lower-segment transverse uterine incision (curve technique) offers many advantages over the vertical uterine incision. Less blood loss, greater ease of repair, less omental and bowel adhesion, less likelihood of tearing into the cervix and vagina, and less likelihood of rupturing along the incision line in future pregnancies are all advantages of the transverse uterine incision. The vertical incision is less likely to tear into the uterine vessels, and it does offer the advantage of more room, if necessary, for the abnormal lie of the fetus.

227. The answer is d. *(Cunningham, 20/e, pp 746–754.)* The patient described in the question presents with a classic history for abruption—that is, the sudden onset of abdominal pain accompanied by bleeding. Physical examination reveals a firm, tender uterus with frequent contractions, which confirms the diagnosis. The fact that a clot forms within 4 min suggests that coagulopathy is not present. Because abruption is often accompanied by hemorrhaging, it is important that appropriate fluids (i.e., lactated Ringer solution and whole blood) be administered immediately to stabilize the mother's circulation. Cesarean section may be necessary in the case of a severe abruption, but only when fetal distress is evident or delivery is unlikely to be accomplished vaginally. Internal monitoring equipment should provide an early warning that the fetus is compromised. The internal uterine catheter provides pressure recordings, which are important if oxytocin stimulation is necessary. Generally, however, patients with abruptio placentae are contracting vigorously and do not need oxytocin.

228–230. The answers are 228-d, 229-b, 230-a. *(Cunningham, 20/e, pp 418–419.)* A woman who has been dilated 9 cm for 3 h is experiencing a secondary arrest in labor. The deteriorating fetal condition (as evidenced, for example, by late decelerations and falling scalp pH) dictates immediate delivery. A forceps rotation would be inappropriate because the cervix is not fully dilated. Cesarean section would be the safest and most expeditious method. Classic cesarean section is rarely used now because of greater blood loss and a higher incidence in subsequent pregnancies of rupture of the scar prior to labor. The best procedure would be a low transverse cesarean section. According to some studies, 25% of twins are diagnosed at the time of delivery. Although sonography or radiography can diagnose multiple gestation early in pregnancy, these methods are not used routinely in all medical centers. The second twin is probably the only remaining situation where internal version is permissible. Although some obstetricians might perform a cesarean section for a second twin presenting as a footling or shoulder, fetal bradycardia dictates that immediate delivery be done, and internal podalic version is the quickest procedure. A transverse lie is undeliverable vaginally. One treatment option is to do nothing and hope that the lie will be longitudinal by the time labor commences. The only other appropriate maneuver would be to perform an external cephalic version. This maneuver should be done in the hospital, with monitoring of the fetal heart. If the version is successful and the cervix is ripe, it might be best to take advantage of the favorable vertex position by rupturing the membranes at that point and inducing labor.

231–233. The answers are 231-b, 232-c, 233-e. *(Cunningham, 20/e, pp 424–426.)* The multiparous patient is in prolonged latent phase, characterized by painful uterine contractions without significant progression in cervical dilatation. Prolongation of latent phase is defined as 20 h in nulliparas and 14 h in multiparas. The diagnosis of this category of uterine dysfunction is difficult and is made in many cases only in retrospect. Only rarely is there need to resort to oxytocic agents or to cesarean section. The recommended management is meperidine (Demerol), 100 mg intramuscularly; this will allow most patients to rest and wake up in active labor. About 10% of patients will wake up without contractions and the diagnosis of false labor will be made. Only about 5% of patients will wake up after meperidine in the same state of contractions without progression. Epidural block may lead to abnormal labor patterns and to delay of descent of the presenting part. In the latter situation, protracted labor is associated with hypotonic uterine dysfunction, a condition that may have been exacerbated by the epidural block. If not contraindicated by other factors (e.g., uterine scar), augmentation of labor by intravenous oxytocin is the treatment of choice in this situation. The patient with arrest of descent and secondary arrest of dilation has adequate uterine contractions. Thus, there is no reason to attempt to augment these contractions by oxytocin. The small-framed mother and the relatively large fetus may suggest cephalopelvic disproportion (CPD). Arrest disorders, common in CPD, and the absence of head engagement despite cervical dilatation also support this diagnosis. The safest way to deliver such a baby would be cesarean section. Early decelerations, which are not depicted in these tracings, occur before the onset of the contraction and represent a vagal response to increased intracranial pressure from uterine pressure on the fetal head.

234–237. The answers are 234-d, 235-a, 236-c, 237-d. (*Cunningham, 20/e, pp 379–399.*) Pudendal block is perhaps the most common form of anesthesia used for vaginal delivery. It provides adequate pain relief for episiotomy, spontaneous delivery, forceps delivery, or vacuum extraction. The success of a pudendal block depends on a clear understanding of the anatomy of the pudendal nerve and its surroundings. Complications (vaginal hematomas, retropsoas, or pelvic abscesses) are quite rare. Paracervical block was a popular form of anesthesia for the first stage of labor until it was implicated in several fetal deaths. It has been shown that paracervical block was associated with fetal bradycardia in 25% to 35% of cases, probably the response to rapid uptake of the drug from the highly vascular paracervical space with a resultant reduction of uteroplacental blood flow. Death in some cases was related to direct injection of the local anesthetic into the fetus. Low spinal anesthesia (saddle block) provides prompt and adequate relief for spontaneous and instrument-assisted delivery. The local anesthetic is injected at the level of the L4–L5 interspace with the patient sitting; although this method is intended to anesthetize the "saddle area," the level of anesthesia may reach sometimes as high as T10. Hypotension and a decrease in uteroplacental perfusion are common results of the profound sympathetic blockade caused by spinal anesthesia. Epidural anesthesia provides effective pain relief for the first and second stages of labor and for delivery. It may be associated with late decelerations suggestive of uteroplacental insufficiency in as many as 20% of cases, but the frequency of this complication may be reduced by prehydration of the mother and by avoiding the supine position. Epidural block appears to lengthen the second stage of labor and is associated with an increased need for augmentation of labor with oxytocin and for instrument-assisted delivery. In experienced hands, however, epidural anesthesia has an excellent safety record.

LACTATION, PUERPERIUM, AND BEHAVIORAL, ETHICAL, AND LEGAL PROBLEMS

Questions

DIRECTIONS: Each item below contains a question or incomplete statement followed by suggested responses. Select the **one best** response to each question.

Items 238–239

A 24-year-old primigravid woman, who is intent on breast feeding, decides upon a home delivery. Immediately after the birth of a 4.1-kg (9-lb) infant, the patient bleeds massively from extensive vaginal and cervical lacerations. She is brought to the nearest hospital in shock. Over 2 h, 9 units of blood are transfused, and the patient's blood pressure returns to a reasonable level. A hemoglobin value the next day is 7.5 g/dL, and 3 units of packed red blood cells are given.

238. The most likely late sequela to consider in this woman would be

a. Hemochromatosis
b. Stein-Leventhal syndrome
c. Sheehan syndrome
d. Simmonds syndrome
e. Cushing syndrome

239. Development of the sequela could be evident as early as

a. 6 h postpartum
b. 1 wk postpartum
c. 1 mo postpartum
d. 6 mo postpartum
e. 1 year postpartum

240. Puerperal fever from breast engorgement

a. Appears in less than 5% of postpartum women
b. Appears 3 to 4 days after the development of lacteal secretion
c. Is almost painless
d. Rarely exceeds 37.8°C (99.8°F)
e. Is less severe and less common if lactation is suppressed

241. A 33-year-old worries about her ability to lactate. Which of the following can interfere with normal lactation?

a. Human placental lactogen
b. Rising progesterone
c. Insulin
d. Thyroid hormones
e. Falling estrogen

242. In the mother, suckling leads to which of the following responses?

a. Decrease of oxytocin
b. Increase of prolactin inhibitory factor
c. Increase of hypothalamic dopamine
d. Increase of hypothalamic prolactin
e. Increase of luteinizing hormone–releasing factor

243. Which of the following statements regarding the postpartum development of pulmonary embolism (PE) is true?

a. It is a relatively uncommon phenomenon with an incidence of about 1:5000
b. In most cases, the classic triad of hemoptysis, pleuritic chest pain, and dyspnea suggests the diagnosis
c. A mismatch in ventilation-perfusion scan is pathognomonic of PE
d. The most common finding at physical examination is a pleuritic friction rub

244. Septic pelvic thrombophlebitis may be characterized by which of the following statements?

a. It usually involves both the iliofemoral and ovarian veins
b. Antimicrobial therapy is usually ineffective
c. Fever spikes are rare
d. It is usually associated with fever without pain or palpable masses
e. Vena caval thrombosis may accompany either ovarian or iliofemoral thrombophlebitis

245. True statements regarding postpartum depression include which of the following?

a. A history of depression is not a risk factor for developing postpartum depression
b. Prenatal preventive intervention for patients at high risk for postpartum depression is best managed alone by a mental health professional
c. Young, multiparous patients are at highest risk
d. Postpartum depression is a self-limiting process that lasts for a maximum of 3 mo
e. About 10% to 12% of women develop postpartum depression

246. A 30-year-old has adverse psychological reactions following hysterectomy. Which of the following is a high-risk factor for development of adverse psychologic responses to gynecologic surgery?

a. Age more than 35
b. Multiparity
c. Prior psychiatric history
d. Proven surgical pathology
e. Less than 12 years of formal education

247. Clinical features of anorexia nervosa include

a. Oily skin
b. Hyperthermia
c. Lethargy
d. Diarrhea
e. Increased incidence of past sexual abuse

248. True statements regarding rape, incest, and abuse include which of the following?

a. Most rape victims are attractive women between 20 and 30 years of age
b. The chance that pregnancy will occur as a result of a rape episode is estimated to be about 25%
c. Approximately 2% to 4% of children are involved in incestual activity
d. Most cases of the sexual abuse of a child involve family members
e. Boys are more likely to be abused than girls

249. The ovaries of an infant at birth contain oocytes that have progressed to

a. Prophase of the first meiotic division
b. Formation of oogonia
c. Maturation
d. Anaphase of the second meiotic division

250. True statements about lesbians include that

a. The great majority of lesbians would like to have children
b. Their behavior is associated with an abnormal hormonal state
c. They have been found to have different personality characteristics from other women
d. The great majority of lesbians are quite open in telling their physicians about their lesbianism
e. Lesbians who do not inform their physicians of their situation refrain out of fear of jeopardizing their medical care

251. A 46-year-old woman presents with depression, urinary urgency, night sweats, and headaches. On examination she is found to be anovulatory. The most likely diagnosis is

a. Psychosomatic disorder
b. Manic depression
c. Urinary tract infection
d. Tuberculosis with renal involvement
e. Menopause

252. A postpartum woman has acute puerperal mastitis. Which of the following statements is true?

a. The initial treatment is penicillin
b. The source of the infection is usually the infant's gastrointestinal (GI) tract
c. Frank abscesses may develop and require drainage
d. The most common offending organism is *Escherichia coli*
e. The symptoms include lethargy

253. A 22-year-old woman, gravida 3, para 2 (one abortion), is brought to the hospital because she states she has been raped by a 35-year-old man whom she knows to have had a vasectomy 2 years ago. Both persons have an A-positive blood type. Which of the following would be most useful to the victim in the prosecution of this case?

a. Accurate description of the introitus
b. Smear for sperm from the cervix
c. Vaginal washings for acid phosphatase
d. Specific typing of vaginal washings
e. Examination of her pubic hair

254. True statements concerning infants born to mothers with active tuberculosis include which of the following?

a. The risk of active disease during the first year of life may approach 90% without prophylaxis
b. Bacille Calmette-Guérin (BCG) vaccination of the newborn infant without evidence of active disease is not appropriate
c. Future ability for tuberculin skin testing is lost after BCG administration to the newborn
d. Neonatal infection is most likely acquired by aspiration of infected amniotic fluid
e. Congenital infection is common despite therapy

255. A 21-year-old has difficulty voiding 6 h postpartum. The least likely cause is which of the following?

a. Preeclampsia
b. Infusion of oxytocin after delivery
c. Vulvar hematoma
d. Urethral trauma
e. Use of general anesthesia

256. Breast feeding can be encouraged despite which of the following conditions?

a. Maternal hepatitis B
b. Maternal reduction mammoplasty with transplantation of the nipples
c. Maternal acute puerperal mastitis
d. Maternal treatment with lithium carbonate
e. Maternal treatment with tetracyclines

Items 257–258

A woman develops endometritis after a cesarean section has been performed. She is treated with penicillin and gentamicin but fails to respond.

257. Which of the following bacteria is resistant to these antibiotics and is likely to be responsible for this woman's infection?

a. *Proteus mirabilis*
b. *Bacteroides fragilis*
c. *Escherichia coli*
d. α streptococci
e. Anaerobic streptococci

258. The treatment of choice for this woman's condition would be

a. Polymyxin
b. Ampicillin
c. Cephalothin
d. Vancomycin
e. Clindamycin

259. A 23-year-old woman (gravida 2, para 2) calls her physician 7 days postpartum because she is concerned that she is still bleeding from the vagina. It would be appropriate to tell this woman that it is normal for bloody lochia to last up to

a. 2 days
b. 5 days
c. 8 days
d. 11 days
e. 14 days

260. A 22-year-old gravida 1, para 0 has just undergone a spontaneous vaginal delivery. As the placenta is being delivered, an inverted uterus prolapses out of the vagina. The maneuver most likely to exacerbate the situations would be to

a. Immediately finish delivering the placenta by removing it from the inverted uterus
b. Call for immediate assistance from other medical personnel
c. Obtain intravenous access and give lactated Ringer solution
d. Apply pressure to the fundus with the palm of the hand and fingers in the direction of the long axis of the vagina
e. Have the anesthesiologist administer halothane anesthesia for uterine relaxation

261. The intramuscular administration of RH_0 immunoglobulin is contraindicated in which of the following situations?

a. After a spontaneous abortion in an Rh-negative, nonsensitized woman
b. In all Rh-negative, nonsensitized women at 28 to 32 wk gestation
c. In all Rh-negative, nonsensitized women within 72 h of the birth of an Rh-positive infant
d. After an episode of uterine bleeding in an Rh-negative, nonsensitized woman
e. After amniocentesis in an Rh-negative, sensitized woman

262. Which of the following potential treatments for use in the initial care of late postpartum hemorrhage would be contraindicated?

a. Methylergonovine maleate (Methergine)
b. Oxytocin injection (Pitocin)
c. Ergonovine maleate (Ergotrate)
d. Prostaglandins
e. Dilation and curettage

263. Following a vaginal delivery, a woman develops a fever, lower abdominal pain, and uterine tenderness. She is alert, and her blood pressure and urine output are good. Large gram-positive rods suggestive of clostridia are seen in a smear of the cervix. Which of the following is most closely tied to a decision to proceed with hysterectomy?

a. Close observation for renal failure or hemolysis
b. Immediate radiographic examination for hydrosalpinx
c. High-dose antibiotic therapy
d. Fever of 103°C
e. Gas gangrene

264. Which of the following goes beyond what the federal Patient Self-Determination Act requires hospitals to do for all patients admitted?

a. Provide all adults with information about their right to accept or refuse treatment if life-threatening conditions arise
b. State the institution's policy on advance directives
c. Not discriminate in care given on the basis of patients' wishes
d. Require assignment of donor organs
e. Allow patients to decide who has the right to make decisions for them

265. A 31-year-old, gravida 3, para 3 Jehovah's Witness begins to bleed heavily 2 days after a cesarean section. She refuses transfusion and says that she would rather die than receive any blood or blood products. You personally feel that you cannot watch her die and do nothing. Appropriate actions that you can take under these circumstances include

a. Telling the patient to find another physician who will care for her
b. Transfusing her forcibly
c. Letting her die, giving only supportive care
d. Getting a court order and transfusing
e. Having the patient's husband sign a release to forcibly transfuse her

266. Which of the following is beyond what a plaintiff must prove in a malpractice action in establishing the standard of care?

a. A doctor-patient relationship was established
b. The defendant owed a duty to the patient
c. The defendant breached a duty to the patient
d. The breach caused damage to the plaintiff
e. The duty is to give the best care possible in the given field

267. A 27-year-old woman who has previously received no prenatal care presents at term. On ultrasound she has a placenta previa, but she refuses a cesarean section for any reason. Important points to consider in her management include

a. The obstetrician's obligation to the supposedly normal fetus supersedes the obligation to the healthy mother
b. The inclusion of several people involved in this complex situation raises the legal risk to the physician
c. Child abuse statutes require the physician to get a court order to force a cesarean section
d. Court-ordered cesarean sections have almost always been determined to achieve the best management
e. A hospital ethics committee should be convened to evaluate the situation

268. In which of the following situations should a court refuse to overturn a living will?

a. At the patient's request, even if he or she is delirious
b. If the patient is pregnant
c. If it has been many years since the signing
d. To allow an organ recipient 1 mo to obtain a donated organ
e. If there is testimony that the patient has changed his or her mind but did not revoke the will

LACTATION, PUERPERIUM, AND BEHAVIORAL, ETHICAL, AND LEGAL PROBLEMS

Answers

238–239. The answers are 238-c, 239-b. *(Cunningham, 20/e, pp 4, 538, 763, 1235.)* A disadvantage of home delivery is the lack of facilities to control postpartum hemorrhage. The woman described in the question delivered a large baby, suffered multiple soft tissue injuries, and went into shock, needing 9 units of blood by the time she reached the hospital. Sheehan syndrome seems a likely possibility in this woman. This syndrome of anterior pituitary necrosis related to obstetric hemorrhage can be diagnosed by 1 wk postpartum, as lactation fails to commence normally. Although many modern women choose hormonal therapy to prevent lactation, the woman described in the question was intent on breast feeding and so would not have received suppressant. She therefore could have been expected to begin lactation at the usual time. Other symptoms of Sheehan syndrome include amenorrhea, atrophy of the breasts, and loss of thyroid and adrenal function. The other presented choices for late sequelae are rather farfetched. Hemochromatosis would not be expected to occur in this healthy young woman, especially since she did not receive prolonged transfusions. Cushing, Simmonds, and Stein-Leventhal syndromes are not known to be related to postpartum hemorrhage. It is important to note that home delivery is not a predisposing factor to postpartum hemorrhage.

240. The answer is e. *(James, 2/e, pp 766–770.)* Puerperal fever from breast engorgement is relatively uncommon, affecting 13% to 18% of postpartum women. It appears 24 to 48 h following initiation of lacteal secretion and it ranges from 38 to 39°C (100.4 to 102.2°F). Pain is an early and common symptom. Treatment consists of breast support, ice packs, and pain relievers. The incidence and severity of breast engorgement are lower if treatment is given for suppression of lactation.

241. The answer is b. (*James, 2/e, pp 766–770.*) A prerequisite for lactation is a fully developed mammary gland. In pregnant women, placental lactogen can substitute for pituitary prolactin and growth hormone. The metabolic hormones insulin and thyroxine are themselves without lactogenic effect, but play a permissive role in this process. Thyroid hormones selectively enhance the secretion of lactalbumin. Estrogen and progesterone, which have a synergistic effect on mammogenesis, inhibit the lactogenic effect of prolactin, and their withdrawal is necessary before initiation of lactation.

242. The answer is d. (*Cunningham, 20/e, pp 536–537.*) The normal sequence of events triggered by suckling is as follows: through a response of the central nervous system, dopamine is decreased in the hypothalamus. Dopamine suppression decreases production of prolactin inhibitory factor (PIF), which normally travels through a portal system to the pituitary gland; because PIF production is decreased, production of prolactin by the pituitary is increased. At this time, the pituitary also releases oxytocin, which causes milk to be expressed from the alveoli into the lactiferous ducts. Suckling suppresses the production of luteinizing hormone–releasing factor and, as a result, acts as a mild contraceptive (because the midcycle surge of luteinizing hormone does not occur).

243. The answer is a. (*Cunningham, 20/e, pp 1114–1116.*) The reported incidence of postpartum pulmonary embolism (PE) is 1:2700 to 1:7000. The classic triad—hemoptysis, pleuritic chest pain, and dyspnea—appears only in 20% of cases. The most common sign on physical examination is tachypnea (>16 breaths/min). Ventilation-perfusion scans with large perfusion defects and ventilation mismatches support the putative diagnosis of PE, but this finding can also be seen with atelectasis or other disorders of lung aeration. To confirm the diagnosis in doubtful cases, there may be a need for pulmonary angiography. Conversely, a normal ventilation-perfusion scan suggests that massive PE is not the etiology of the clinical symptoms.

244. The answer is e. (*Cunningham, 20/e, pp 556–558.*) Septic thrombophlebitis may involve either the iliofemoral or the ovarian vein but rarely involves both sites in the same patient. Vena caval thrombosis may follow either ovarian or iliofemoral phlebitis. The clinical presentation is that of a pelvic infection with pain and fever. Following antimicrobial therapy, clinical symptoms usually resolve, but fever spikes may continue. Commonly, patients do not appear clinically ill. The diagnosis is made by computerized tomography (CT) or by magnetic resonance imaging (MRI). Before these diagnostic modalities were available, the heparin challenge test was advocated—lysis of fever after intravenous administration of heparin was accepted as diagnostic for pelvic thrombophlebitis. It seems, however, that clinical symptoms may respond to antimicrobials alone, despite evidence of pelvic thrombophlebitis on MRI, and the febrile course is not changed significantly by administration of heparin.

245. The answer is e. (*Cunningham, 20/e, pp 1265–1268.*) Patients at high risk for postpartum depression often have histories of depression or postpartum depression. They are more likely to be primiparous or older; they may have had a long interval between pregnancies or an unplanned pregnancy or be without a supportive partner. Prenatal intervention must include the obstetric team, with family or peer support when possible. Postpartum depression is variable in duration, but occasionally will not resolve without hospitalization, therapy, or medication.

246. The answer is c. (*Mishell, 3/e, pp 753–755.*) Risks for adverse psychologic responses to gynecologic surgery include age <35, nulliparity, less than high school education, and absence of active surgical pathology. The presurgical period is the most important time to sort out these factors and take necessary steps. An ideal treatment team to deal with these problems would include the gynecologist, a psychiatrist, and a nurse.

247. The answer is e. (*Curtis, 5/e, p 245.*) Anorexia nervosa, which occurs in approximately 1 per 100,000 patients, is seen almost exclusively in females. The patients tend to be hyperactive, suffer from constipation, and have amenorrhea, coarse, dry skin, a distortion of body self-image, and a higher than average incidence of past sexual abuse. Mortality with anorexia nervosa has been reported to be as high as 9%, mostly secondary to cardiac arrhythmias.

248. The answer is d. (*Mishell, 3/e, pp 197–202.*) Sexual assault happens to people of all ages. The mentally and physically handicapped and the very old are particularly susceptible. Victims of rape should always be treated as victims and at no time should the implication of guilt be applied to them. Psychologic reaction to rape includes two phases: an immediate phase of paralysis of the coping mechanisms, usually lasting hours or days, followed by a more prolonged period of reorganization that may last months to years. The victim's menstrual history, birth control regimen, and known pregnancy status should be assessed at the initial examination. In the experience of most sexual assault centers, the chance that pregnancy will occur as a result of sexual assault is quite small and has been estimated to be approximately 2% to 4% for victims having a single unprotected coitus. If the patient has been exposed at midcycle, the risk would obviously be higher. "Morning after" prophylaxis using high-dose estrogens or oral contraceptives should be offered to unprotected rape victims.

About 10% of all abused children are also sexually abused. Although the crime is underreported, it is estimated that about 336,000 children are sexually abused each year in the United States. Incestual activity may be experienced by as many as 15% to 25% of women and 12% of men. A family member is the sexual abuser of a child in about 80% of cases. Father-daughter incest accounts for about 75% of reported cases. A brother-sister relationship may be the most common type of incest but is reported less frequently.

249. The answer is a. (*Reece, 2/e, pp 4–5.*) Evidence of nuclear maturation is first seen at about 15 wk gestation. The oogonia are transformed to oocytes as they enter the first meiotic division and arrest in prophase. The second meiotic division is not completed until fertilization.

250. The answer is e. (*Mishell, 3/e, pp 182–183.*) Studies on adult sexual behavior have shown that it is the result of interactions of biologic, psychologic, developmental, and sociologic factors. Studies on lesbian women have been nondiagnostic in terms of finding either altered hormonal states or personality traits that differ from those of other women. In separate surveys, 49% of lesbians stated that they had considered having children, and the same number stated that they had told their physicians of their lesbianism. Of those lesbians who did not inform their doctors of their sexual orientation, most stated that they did not because of fear of jeopardizing their medical care.

251. The answer is e. (*Mishell, 3/e, p 1159.*) The symptoms described in the question are common symptoms of menopause. They all result primarily from estrogen withdrawal, and most can be reversed by estrogen therapy. *Climacteric* is actually a better word for this complex of symptoms because the menopause is technically the instant at which menses ceases.

252. The answer is c. *(Ransom, 2000, pp 172–174.)* Puerperal mastitis may be subacute but is often characterized by chills, fever, and tachycardia. If undiagnosed, it may progress to suppurative mastitis with abscess formation that requires drainage. The most common offending organism is *Staphylococcus aureus,* which is probably transmitted from the infant's nose and throat. This in turn is most likely acquired from personnel in the nursery. At times, epidemics of suppurative mastitis have developed. A penicillinase-resistant antibiotic is the initial treatment of choice.

253. The answer is c. *(Mishell, 3/e, pp 198–202.)* Although all the procedures mentioned in the question can be helpful in establishing a case of rape in most situations, the expected lack of sperm and the matching blood types in the situation presented would limit their value in this case. Only the finding of 50 units/mL or more of acid phosphatase in this woman's vagina could be taken as evidence of ejaculation. Her introitus probably would not be injured because of her parity. Foreign pubic hair might only indicate close contact.

254. The answer is c. *(Cunningham, 20/e, p 946.)* The goal of management in the infant born to a mother with active tuberculosis is prevention of early neonatal infection. Congenital infection, acquired either by a hematogenous route or by aspiration of infected amniotic fluid, is rare. Most neonatal infections are acquired by postpartum maternal contact. The risk of active disease during the first year of life may approach 50% if prophylaxis is not instituted. BCG vaccination and daily isonicotinic acid hydrazide (isoniazid, INH) therapy are both acceptable means of therapy. BCG vaccination may be easier because it requires only one injection; however, the ability to perform future tuberculin skin testing is lost.

255. The answer is a. *(Cunningham, 20/e, pp 258, 262, 265.)* An inability to void often leads to the diagnosis of a vulvar hematoma. Such hematomas are often large enough to apply pressure on the urethra. Pain from urethral lacerations is another reason women have difficulty voiding after delivery. Both general anesthesia, which temporarily disturbs neural control of the bladder, and oxytocin, which has an antidiuretic effect, can lead to an overdistended bladder and an inability to void. In this case an indwelling catheter should be inserted and left in for at least 24 h to allow recovery of normal bladder tone and sensation. Preeclampsia often leads to edema that generally leads to diuresis postpartum.

256. The answer is c. (*James, 2/e, pp 766–770.*) There are very few contraindications to breast feeding. In acute viral infections, such as hepatitis B, there is the possibility of transmitting the virus in the milk. Most medications taken by the mother enter into breast milk, usually in concentrations similar to or less than those in maternal plasma. Breast feeding is inadvisable when the mother is being treated with antimitotic drugs, tetracyclines, diagnostic or therapeutic radioactive substances, or lithium carbonate. Acute puerperal mastitis may be managed quite successfully while the mother continues to breast feed. Reduction mammoplasty with autotransplantation of the nipple simply makes breast feeding impossible.

257–258. The answers are 257-b, 258-e. (*Gleicher, 3/e, pp 584–594.*) Infections caused by *Bacteroides fragilis*, a gram-negative anaerobic bacillus, are a significant obstetric problem. Not only is the organism resistant to many commonly used antibiotics (including penicillin and gentamicin), but it is difficult to isolate, culture, and identify as well. The high incidence of gynecologic and obstetric *B. fragilis* infections may be due to the pathogen's predominance among the anaerobic bacteria of the lower bowel. Although the other organisms listed in the question also can cause postpartum infection, they are sensitive to antibiotic therapy with penicillin and gentamicin. Clindamycin is the most effective antibiotic for treating women who have bacteroidosis. Chloramphenicol and tetracycline are alternative choices for antibiotic therapy in nonpregnant women; however, tetracycline-resistant strains of *B. fragilis* may be emerging. Lincomycin and erythromycin can also be effective in the management of affected women.

259. The answer is e. (*Cunningham, 20/e, pp 540, 551.*) Bloody lochia can persist for up to 2 wk without indicating an underlying pathology; however, if bleeding continues beyond 2 wk, it may indicate placental site subinvolution, retention of small placental fragments, or both. At this point, appropriate diagnostic and therapeutic measures should be initiated. The physician should first estimate the blood loss and then perform a pelvic examination in search of uterine subinvolution or tenderness. Excessive bleeding or tenderness should lead the physician to suspect retained placental fragments or endometritis. A larger than expected but otherwise asymptomatic uterus supports the diagnosis of subinvolution.

260. The answer is a. (*Hankins, pp 273–279.*) If attached, the placenta is not removed until the infusion systems are operational, fluids are being given, and anesthesia (preferably halothane) has been administered. To remove the placenta before this time increases hemorrhage. As soon as the uterus is restored to its normal configuration, the anesthetic agent used to provide relaxation is stopped and simultaneously oxytocin is started to contract the uterus.

261. The answer is e. (*Queenan, 4/e, pp 399–409.*) Prior to the use of Rh_0 immunoglobulin in the nonsensitized Rh-negative woman who delivered an Rh-positive infant, the isoimmunization rate was about 10%. The use of Rh_0 immunoglobulin is also recommended in Rh-negative, nonsensitized women after abortion, molar pregnancy, ectopic pregnancy, amniocentesis, or vaginal bleeding in pregnancy. Nearly 1.8% of Rh-negative women become sensitized during the third trimester. Administration of Rh_0 immunoglobulin at 28 to 32 wk in the Rh-negative, nonsensitized woman has decreased the rate of sensitization to 0.07%.

262. The answer is e. (*Cunningham, 20/e, pp 760–779.*) Uterine hemorrhage after the first postpartum week is most often the result of retained placental fragments or subinvolution of the placental site. Curettage may do more harm than benefit by stimulating increased bleeding. Initial therapy should be aimed at decreasing the bleeding by stimulating uterine contractions with the use of Pitocin, Methergine, or Ergotrate. Prostaglandins could also be used in this setting.

263. The answer is e. (*Cunningham, 20/e, pp 1065–1069.*) Clostridia can be seen in 5% to 10% of pelvic cultures. When the organism is found, appropriate antibiotic therapy (e.g., with penicillin) and close observation for gas gangrene, hemolysis, and renal failure are in order. Presumed identification on the basis of gram stain alone or the presence of mild infection without signs of sepsis or extrauterine involvement is not reason enough to proceed to hysterectomy.

264. The answer is d. (*Scott, 8/e, pp 939–954.*) Hospitals must now inform patients about their rights to accept or refuse terminal care. Such information has to be documented in the patient's chart. The patient has the option to make a clear assignment of who can make decisions if the patient cannot. Patients are not required to allow organ donation.

265. The answer is c. (*American College of Obstetricians and Gynecologists, 1987.*) Determination of ethical conduct in doctor-patient relationships can sometimes be very difficult for the physician who is confronted with a patient's autonomy in making a decision that the physician finds incomprehensible. However, the autonomy of the patient who is oriented and alert must be respected even if it means in effect that the patient is committing suicide. The obtaining of court orders to transfuse an adult against his or her will is almost never an acceptable option and leads to a tremendous "slippery slope" of the doctor's control of the patient's behavior. A patient's spouse also does not have legal authority to make decisions for the patient if the patient is competent, awake, and alert. The situation is different if there is a child involved, when societal interests can occasionally override parental autonomy. It would be inappropriate for a physician to abandon a patient without obtaining suitable coverage from another qualified physician. Transfusing forcibly is assault and battery; thus, in this case, the physician must adhere to the patient's wishes and, if need be, let her die.

266. The answer is e. (*Ransom, 2000, pp 786–792.*) Negligence law governs conduct and embraces acts of both commission and omission, i.e., what a person did or failed to do. In general the law expects all persons to conduct themselves in a fashion that does not expose others to an unreasonable risk of harm. In a fiduciary relationship such as the physician-patient relationship, the physician is held to a higher standard of behavior because of the imbalance of knowledge. In general, the real gist of negligence is not carelessness or ineptitude, but rather how unreasonable the risk of harm the patient was exposed to by the physician's action. Thus physicians are held accountable to a standard of care that asks the question, "What would the reasonable physician do under this specific set of circumstances?" One is not held accountable to the level of the leading experts in any given field, but rather the prevailing standards among average practitioners. When a doctor-patient relationship is established, the defendant owes a duty to the patient. If the defendant breaches that duty—i.e., acts in a way that is inconsistent with the standard of care and that can be shown to have caused damage directly to the patient (proximate damage)—then the physician may be held liable for compensation.

267. The answer is e. *(Gleicher, 3/e, pp 206–210.)* When confronted by a complex situation in which there are conflicting values and rights, getting the most people involved is the best approach to reduce risk and to come up with the best, most defensible answer under the current circumstances. The obstetrician should employ whatever departmental or hospital resources are available. A standing ethics committee or an ad hoc committee to deal with such complex situations is often available and will minimize the ultimate medicolegal problems that can ensue when bad outcomes seem likely. The obstetrician must further recognize that he or she has two patients, but that it is not clear, nor is it legislated, whose interests take priority. However, general ethical opinion is that the mother generally should come first. Most court-ordered cesarean sections have been performed on patients who were estranged from the medical system, and this sets a very bad precedent for further state intervention in doctor-patient relationships and maternal rights. Child abuse statutes do not at this point require a court order to force a cesarean section even for a healthy fetus, and a court order would almost never be appropriate.

268. The answer is d. *(Scott, 8/e, pp 939–954.)* Living wills represent the chance for patients to declare their wishes in advance of situations in which they become no longer competent to do so. They are revocable by the patient at any time and are automatically invalid if the patient is pregnant, as another being is involved. Living wills can be set aside if a long period has elapsed since their drafting and the wishes are not known to be current. Also, there is the potential for conflict if the patient has signed a donor card and prolongation of life would be needed to carry out those wishes. Generally, such action would not be honored unless relatively expeditious arrangements were possible.

GYNECOLOGY

ANATOMY, PUBERTY, MENSTRUATION, AND MENOPAUSE

Questions

DIRECTIONS: Each item below contains a question or incomplete statement followed by suggested responses. Select the **one best** response to each question.

269. You see five postmenopausal patients in the clinic. Each patient has one of the conditions listed below, and each patient wishes to begin hormone replacement therapy today. Which patient would you start on therapy at the time of this visit?

a. Mild essential hypertension
b. Liver disease with abnormal liver function tests
c. Malignant melanoma
d. Undiagnosed genital tract bleeding
e. Treated Stage III endometrial cancer

270. Which of the following screening tools for osteoporosis is currently recommended for all menopausal women?

a. Spinal x-ray
b. Dual-energy x-ray absorptiometry
c. Single-photon absorptiometry
d. Dual-photon absorptiometry
e. Periodic health maintenance visits

271. The first evidence of pubertal development in the female is usually

a. Onset of menarche
b. Appearance of breast buds
c. Appearance of axillary and pubic hair
d. Onset of growth spurt

272. A 9-year-old girl presents for evaluation of regular vaginal bleeding. History reveals thelarche at age 7 and adrenarche at age 8. The most common cause of this condition in girls is

a. Idiopathic
b. Gonadal tumors
c. McCune-Albright syndrome
d. Hypothyroidism
e. Tumors of the central nervous system

273. Estrogen replacement therapy has been shown to do which of the following?

a. Increase the risk of ovarian cancer
b. Provide protection against coronary heart disease
c. Increase levels of low-density lipoprotein
d. Decrease levels of high-density lipoprotein
e. Prevent rheumatoid arthritis

274. Major endocrine changes occur in menopause. Which of the following is a true statement concerning menopause?

a. The ovary secretes more testosterone than previously
b. Estrone is produced by peripheral conversion from testosterone
c. Circulating androstenedione is decreased by 90%
d. Follicle-stimulating hormone (FSH) levels rise after cessation of menses
e. Estradiol is the major estrogen produced in adipose tissue

275. A 50-year-old woman is diagnosed with cervical cancer. Which lymph node group would be the first to be involved in metastatic spread of this disease beyond the cervix and uterus in this patient?

a. Common iliac nodes
b. Parametrial nodes
c. External iliac nodes
d. Paracervical or ureteral nodes
e. Paraaortic nodes

276. A 55-year-old woman complains of seborrhea, acne, and mild facial hirsutism since menopause 2 years ago. Her serum androstenedione and estrone levels are moderately elevated. Which of the following is the most likely cause of her condition?

a. Amount of body fat
b. Increased ovarian steroid secretion
c. Increased adrenal steroid secretion
d. Diminished renal steroid elimination
e. Diminished hepatic steroid clearance

277. Which of the following is a true statement regarding the psychological symptoms of the climacteric?

a. They are considerably less important than hormone levels
b. They commonly include insomnia, irritability, frustration, and malaise
c. They are related to a drop in gonadotropin levels
d. They are not affected by environmental factors
e. They are primarily a reaction to the cessation of menstrual flow

278. Osteoporosis is least likely in which of the following women?

a. Asian
b. Caucasian
c. Smokers
d. Those who lead a sedentary lifestyle
e. Obese

279. Which of the following is consistent with a diagnosis of delayed puberty?

a. Breast budding is absent in a 10-year-old girl
b. Menarche is delayed beyond 16 years of age
c. Menarche begins 1 year after breast budding
d. FSH values are less than 20 mIU/mL

280. Which of the following has been identified as an etiologic factor in the majority of women with premenstrual syndrome?

a. Anovulatory cycles
b. Altered prostaglandin levels
c. Altered pituitary hormone levels
d. Altered β-endorphin levels
e. Ovarian function

281. An 18-year-old patient consults you for evaluation of disabling pain with her menstrual periods. The pain has been present since menarche and is accompanied by nausea and headache. History is otherwise unremarkable, and pelvic examination is normal. You diagnose primary dysmenorrhea and recommend initial treatment with which of the following?

a. Ergot derivatives
b. Antiprostaglandins
c. Gonadotropin-releasing hormone (GnRH) analogs
d. Danazol
e. Codeine

282. Normal stature with minimal or absent pubertal development may be seen in

a. Testicular feminization
b. Kallman syndrome
c. Pure gonadal dysgenesis
d. Turner syndrome
e. Intermittent athletic training

283. Medications used in the treatment of idiopathic central precocious puberty include

a. Exogenous gonadotropins
b. Ethinyl estradiol
c. GnRH agonist
d. Clomiphene citrate
e. Conjugated estrogens (e.g., Premarin)

284. Delayed puberty and sexual infantilism associated with hypergonadotropic hypogonadism can be seen in patients with which of the following?

a. Adrenogenital syndrome (testicular feminization)
b. McCune-Albright Syndrome
c. Kallman syndrome
d. Gonadal dysgenesis
e. Müllerian agenesis

285. While evaluating a 30-year-old woman for infertility, you diagnose a bicornuate uterus. You explain to the couple that additional testing is necessary in this woman because of the increased risk of congenital anomalies in which organ system?

a. Skeletal
b. Hematopoetic
c. Urinary
d. Central nervous system
e. Tracheoesophageal

DIRECTIONS: Each group of questions below consists of lettered options followed by numbered items. For each numbered item, select the appropriate lettered option(s). Each lettered option may be used once, more than once, or not at all. **Choose exactly the number of options indicated following each item.**

Items 286–290

For each description below, select the type of sexual precocity with which it is most likely to be associated.

a. True sexual precocity
b. Incomplete sexual precocity
c. Isosexual precocious pseudopuberty
d. Heterosexual precocious pseudopuberty
e. Precocity due to gonadotropin-producing tumors

286. Defined by the presence of virilizing signs in girls (**SELECT 1 PRECOCITY**)

287. Characterized by the presence of premature adrenarche, pubarche, or thelarche (**SELECT 1 PRECOCITY**)

288. Can arise from cranial tumors or hypothyroidism (**SELECT 1 PRECOCITY**)

289. Results from premature activation of the hypothalamic-pituitary system (**SELECT 1 PRECOCITY**)

290. Is frequently caused by ovarian tumors (**SELECT 1 PRECOCITY**)

Items 291–295

For each description that follows, select the blood vessel with which it is most likely to be associated.

a. Uterine vein
b. Right ovarian vein
c. Left ovarian vein
d. Uterine artery
e. Ovarian artery

291. Arises from the anterior branch of the hypogastric artery (**SELECT 1 VESSEL**)

292. Drains into the internal iliac veins (**SELECT 1 VESSEL**)

293. Drains into the inferior vena cava (**SELECT 1 VESSEL**)

294. Arises from the abdominal aorta (**SELECT 1 VESSEL**)

295. Drains into the renal vein (**SELECT 1 VESSEL**)

ANATOMY, PUBERTY, MENSTRUATION, AND MENOPAUSE

Answers

269. The answer is a. (*Speroff 6/e, pp 761–766.*) Absolute contraindications to postmenopausal hormone replacement therapy include the presence of estrogen-dependent tumors (breast or uterus), active thromboembolic disease, undiagnosed genital tract bleeding, active severe liver disease, and malignant melanoma. Past or current history of hypertension, diabetes, or biliary stones does not automatically disqualify a patient for hormone replacement therapy.

270. The answer is e. (*Adashi, pp 1826–1839.*) At the present time, the use of radiologic screening techniques for osteoporosis in all patients is controversial. X-rays will pick up fractures and bone abnormalities but will miss osteoporosis unless a significant amount of bone loss (at least 20% to 30%) is already present. Single-photon absorptiometry is accurate in predicting bone loss in the radius; however, its sensitivity is decreased in the axial skeleton. Dual-photon absorptiometry is more accurate in this regard, while dual-energy x-ray absorptiometry (DEXA) is a sensitive technique with low radiation exposure and patient discomfort. At the present time it is thought that, for women who are reluctant to use estrogen in the menopausal period, dual-photon absorptiometry, quantitative computerized tomography, or DEXA may be used to document rapid bone loss and determine whether the patient is at significant risk for developing fractures. Of these three techniques, DEXA is probably best for clinical use. However, these tests are not screening tools to be used on all menopausal patients, since the cost-effectiveness of screening using these techniques is unproven. Instead, periodic annual examinations are used to identify patients at risk in whom these specific diagnostic tests are then employed.

271. The answer is b. *(Speroff 6/e, pp 386–391. Adashi, pp 76–92.)* In the United States, the appearance of breast buds (thelarche) is usually the first sign of puberty, usually occurring between the ages of 9 and 11 years. This is subsequently followed by the appearance of pubic and axillary hair (adrenarche or pubarche), the adolescent growth spurt, and finally menarche. On average, the sequence of developmental changes requires a period of 4.5 years to complete, with a range of 1.5 to 6 years. The average ages of adrenarche/pubarche and menarche are 11.0 and 12.8 years, respectively. These events are considered to be delayed if thelarche has not occurred by the age of 13, adrenarche has not occurred by the age of 14, or menarche by the age of 16. Girls with delayed sexual development should be fully evaluated for delayed puberty, which includes central, ovarian, systemic, or constitutional causes.

272. The answer is a. *(Speroff 6/e, pp 392–403. Adashi, pp 990–1006.)* In North America, pubertal changes before the age of 8 years in girls and 9 years in boys are regarded as precocious. Although the most common type of precocious puberty in girls is idiopathic, it is essential to ensure close long-term follow-up of these patients to ascertain that there is no serious underlying pathology, such as tumors of the central nervous system or ovary. Only 1% to 2% of patients with precocious puberty have an estrogen-producing ovarian tumor as the causative factor. McCune-Albright syndrome (polyostotic fibrous dysplasia) is also relatively rare and consists of fibrous dysplasia and cystic degeneration of the long bones, sexual precocity, and café au lait spots on the skin. Hypothyroidism is a cause of precocious puberty in some children, making thyroid function tests mandatory in these cases. Tumors of the central nervous system as a cause of precocious puberty occur more commonly in boys than in girls; they are seen in about 11% of girls with precocious puberty.

273. The answer is b. *(Speroff 6/e, pp 730, 765–766.)* Estrogen replacement therapy is useful in the prevention of osteoporosis and in protecting women against atherosclerotic vascular disease including coronary artery disease (angina, nonfatal and fatal myocardial infarction) and cerebrovascular disease. Postmenopausal estrogen users have decreased levels of total and low-density lipoprotein (LDL) and increased levels of high-density lipoprotein (HDL). Triglyceride levels are usually mildly increased in users of estrogen alone. The addition of progestins such as medroxyprogesterone acetate (Provera), recommended in postmenopausal estrogen users who retain their uteruses to counter the proliferative effects of estrogen on the endometrium, can reverse some of these beneficial effects. Postmenopausal estrogen intake has not been shown to significantly increase the risk of ovarian cancer in women. Studies on its relation to breast cancer are more confusing, but at this time use of estrogen does not appear to increase the risk of breast cancer in the majority of postmenopausal women. There is no direct protective or beneficial effect of estrogen on rheumatoid arthritis in postmenopausal women.

274. The answer is a. (*Speroff 6/e, pp 656–660.*) With the population as a whole increasing in age, the problems of the postmenopausal woman are a major public health concern. Significant endocrine changes occur in the perimenopausal and postmenopausal period. In the premenopausal period, estrogen output from the ovary begins to decline. With the loss of central negative feedback, FSH levels begin to rise, despite continued menstrual bleeding. Choice d is therefore incorrect since FSH levels do not rise after cessation of menses, but rather before menses stops. Eventually, there is a 10- to 20-fold increase in circulating FSH levels and a variable increase in luteinizing hormone (LH). Sustained elevation of both hormones is conclusive evidence of ovarian failure. Serum levels of androstenedione decrease by 50%, with the majority of circulating androstenedione produced by the adrenal gland. The postmenopausal ovary, however, secretes more testosterone than does the premenopausal ovary in the first few years after menopause, secondary to gonadotropin stimulation of ovarian stromal tissue. The major source of postmenopausal estrogen is estrone, which is derived from peripheral conversion of androstenedione in the adipose tissue. Virtually all circulating estradiol is the result of peripheral conversion from testosterone, and not secretion from the ovary as in the premenopausal women.

275. The answer is d. (*DiSaia, 5/e, pp 55–62.*) The main routes of spread of cervical cancer include vaginal mucosa, myometrium, paracervical lymphatics, and direct extension into the parametrium. The prevalence of lymph node disease correlates with the stage of malignancy. Primary node groups involved in the spread of cervical cancer include the paracervical, parametrial, obturator, hypogastric, external iliac, and sacral nodes, essentially in that order. Less commonly there is involvement in the common iliac, inguinal, and para-aortic nodes. In stage I, the pelvic nodes are positive in approximately 15% of cases and the para-aortic nodes in 6%. In stage II, pelvic nodes are positive in 28% of cases and para-aortic nodes in 16%. In stage III, pelvic nodes are positive in 47% of cases and para-aortic nodes in 28%.

276. The answer is a. (*Speroff 6/e, pp 658–662.*) Peripheral conversion of androstenedione to estrone in adipose tissue is the major source of estrogens in the postmenopausal woman. The conversion rate and the resulting estrogen levels are thus dependent on the circulating free androgen levels and the amount of body fat. In obese women, higher estrone levels will be found and menopausal symptoms will be less severe and less frequent. These women are also less likely to develop osteoporosis. Especially in obese postmenopausal women, this prolonged and unopposed estrogen stimulation may cause uterine bleeding, endometrial hyperplasia, and adenocarcinoma.

277. The answer is b. (*Ransom 2000, pp 593–598.*) Psychological symptoms during the climacteric occur at a time when much is changing in a women's life. Steroid hormone levels are dropping, and the menses is stopping. However, studies show these two factors to be unrelated to emotional symptoms in most women. Many factors, such as hormonal, environmental, and intrapsychic elements, combine to cause the resulting symptoms of the climacteric such as insomnia, vasomotor instability (hot flushes, hot flashes), emotional lability, and genital tract atrophy with vulvar, vaginal, and urinary symptoms.

278. The answer is e. (*Speroff 6/e, pp 691–707.*) A major menopausal health issue is osteoporosis, which results in fractures of the vertebral bodies, humerus, upper femur, forearm, and ribs. Patients with vertebral fractures will experience back pain, gastrointestinal motility disorders, restrictive pulmonary symptoms, and loss of mobility. There may be a gradual decrease in height as well. Although all races experience osteoporosis, white and Asian women lose bone earlier and at a more rapid rate than black women. Thin women and those who smoke are at increased risk for developing osteoporosis. Physical activity increases the mineral content of bone in postmenopausal women.

279. The answer is b. *(Adashi, pp 1007–1015.)* Significant emotional concerns develop when puberty is delayed. By definition, if breast development has not begun by age 13, delayed puberty should be suspected. Menarche usually follows about 1 to 2 years after the beginning of breast development; if menarche is delayed beyond age 16, delayed puberty should be investigated. Appropriate laboratory tests including circulating pituitary and steroid hormone levels, karyotypic analysis, and central nervous system (CNS) imaging when indicated should be ordered. An FSH value greater than 40 mIU/mL defines hypergonadotropic hypogonadism as a cause of delayed pubertal maturation. Hypergonadotropic hypogonadism is seen in girls with gonadal dysgenesis, such as Turner Syndrome. Since gonadal dysgenesis is a such a common cause of absent pubertal development, hypergonadotropic hypogonadism is frequently—but not invariably—found in these patients.

280. The answer is e. *(Adashi, pp 1636–1647.)* Premenstrual syndrome (PMS) is a cyclic disturbance in which luteal phase symptoms occur followed by a symptom-free interval after menses. The diagnostic criteria also include the absence of other psychiatric or organic pathology and require that the symptom complex interfere in some way with the woman's daily life, such as her work, school, relationships, etc. PMS includes combinations of emotional, behavioral, and physical symptoms, such as headache, breast swelling and tenderness, edema, abdominal pain, abdominal bloating, fatigue, irritability, tension, anxiety, and depression. Most women suffer from only one or a few of the symptoms from the list of over 100 symptoms possibly associated with PMS. While the combination of symptoms present in each patient is unique, that particular combination tends to recur consistently with each cycle in a given patient. PMS can occur in both ovulatory and anovulatory cycles, although it is much more common in ovulatory ones. The cause of the premenstrual symptoms is not known, and many theories have been proposed. Abnormal levels of estrogens and progesterone, hypoglycemia, vitamin deficiency, prostaglandins, and β-endorphins have been implicated. However, no etiologic factor has been identified that appears to be present in a majority of the patients studied. This lack of consistent etiologic findings could reflect either the fact that multiple etiologies cause this syndrome, differences in definition and identification of patients, or some other explanation. One certainty regarding etiology is that ovarian function appears to be necessary for PMS, since the syndrome disappears in postmenopausal women. Treatment is empiric and ranges from diuretics through psychologic support to progesterone support of the luteal phase. The selective serotonin reuptake inhibitors (SSRIs) have recently shown considerable promise in treating women with PMS. In a number of cases, relief of breast symptoms is significant after elimination from the diet of coffee, tea, chocolate, and other products containing caffeine and methylxanthine.

281. The answer is b. (*Scott 8/e, p 613.*) Dysmenorrhea is considered secondary if associated with pelvic disease such as endometriosis, uterine myomas, or pelvic inflammatory disease. Primary dysmenorrhea is associated with a normal pelvic examination and with ovulatory cycles. The pain of dysmenorrhea is usually accompanied by other symptoms—nausea, fatigue, diarrhea, and headache—which may be related to excess of prostaglandin $F_{2\alpha}$. The two major drug therapies effective in dysmenorrhea are oral contraceptives and antiprostaglandins. GnRH analogs are used in several gynecologic conditions, but would not be first-line therapy for primary dysmenorrhea. Similarly, danazol is used for the treatment of endometriosis, and ergot derivatives for hyperprolactinemia. Analgesics such as codeine or narcotics would generally be employed only in very severe cases when no other treatment provides adequate relief. Treatment will reduce the number of women incapacitated by menstrual symptoms to about 10% of those treated. Contrary to past beliefs, psychologic factors play only a minor role in dysmenorrhea.

282. The answer is b. (*Scott 8/e, pp 603–604. Speroff 6/e, pp 404–407.*) Testicular feminization is a syndrome of androgen insensitivity in genetic males, characterized by a normal 46,X genotype, normal female phenotype during childhood, tall stature, and "normal" breast development with absence of axillary and pubic hair. Breast development (gynecomastia) occurs in these males because high levels of circulating testosterone (which cannot act at its receptor) are aromatized to estrogen, which then acts on the breast. The external genitalia develop as those of a female because testosterone cannot masculinize them, while the müllerian structures are absent because of testicular secretion of müllerian-inhibiting factor *in utero*. Gonadal dysgenesis—e.g., 45,X Turner syndrome—is characterized by short stature and absence of pubertal development; in these girls the ovaries are either absent or streak gonads that are nonfunctional. In either case estrogen production is possible, and hence isosexual pubertal development does not occur. Kallman syndrome (hypogonadotropic hypogonadism) should be suspected in patients of normal stature with delayed or absent pubertal development, especially when associated with the classic finding of anosmia. These individuals have a structural defect of the CNS involving the hypothalamus and the olfactory bulbs (located in close proximity to the hypothalamus), such that the hypothalamus does not secrete GnRH in normal pulsatile fashion, if at all. Other causes of minimal or absent pubertal development with normal stature include malnutrition, anorexia nervosa, severe systemic disease, and intensive athletic training, particularly ballet and running.

283. The answer is c. *(Speroff 6/e, pp 401–403.)* Precocious puberty can be treated by agents that reduce gonadotropin levels by exerting negative feedback in the hypothalamic-pituitary axis or that directly inhibit gonadotropin secretion from the pituitary gland. Until about 10 years ago, the greatest experience in the treatment of idiopathic central precocious puberty was with medroxyprogesterone acetate (MPA). MPA was usually administered intramuscularly in a dose of 100 to 200 mg/wk, or orally at 20 to 40 mg/day. Currently, the most effective treatment for central precocious puberty is the use of a long-acting GnRH agonist, such as leurolide (Lupron) and others. These drugs act by downregulating pituitary gonadotropes, eventually decreasing the secretion of FSH and LH, which are inappropriately stimulating the ovaries of these patients. As a result of this induced hypogonadotropic state, ovarian steroids (estrogens, progestins, and androgens) are suppressed back to prepubertal levels, and the precocious pubertal development stops or regresses. During the first 1 or 2 wk of therapy there is a "flare-up" effect of increased gonadotropins and sex steroids, a predicted side effect of these medications. At the time of expected puberty, the GnRH analog is discontinued and the pubertal sequence resumes.

284. The answer is d. *(Speroff 6/e, pp 404–407. Adashi, pp 1008–1015.)* Delayed puberty is a rare condition, usually differentiated into hypergonadotropic (high FSH and LH levels) hypogonadism or hypogonadotropic (low FSH and LH) hypogonadism. The most common cause of hypergonadotropic hypogonadism is gonadal dysgenesis, i.e., the 45,X Turner syndrome. Hypogonadotropic hypogonadism can be seen in patients with hypothalamic-pituitary or constitutional delays in development. Kallmann syndrome presents with amenorrhea, infantile sexual development, low gonadotropins, normal female karyotype, and anosmia (the inability to perceive odors). In addition to those conditions listed above, many other types of medical and nutritional problems can lead to this type of delayed development, e.g., malabsorption, diabetes, regional ileitis, and other chronic illness. Congenital adrenal hyperplasia leads to early pubertal development, although in girls the development is not isosexual (ie., not of the expected sex) and would therefore include hirsutism, clitoromegaly, and other signs of virilization. Complete müllerian agenesis is a condition in which the müllerian ducts either fail to develop or regress early in fetal life. These patients have a blind vaginal pouch and no upper vagina, cervix, or uterus, and they present with primary amenorrhea. However, because ovarian development is not affected, secondary sexual characteristics develop normally despite the absence of menarche, and gonadotropin levels are normal. The McCune-Albright syndrome involves the constellation of precocious puberty, café au lait spots, and polyostotic fibrous dysplasia.

285. The answer is c. _(Speroff 6/e, pp 440–442.)_ Failed fusion of the müllerian ducts can give rise to several types of uterine anomalies, of which bicornuate uterus is a representative type. This condition is associated with a higher risk of obstetric complications, such as an increase in the rate of second-trimester abortion and premature labor. If these pregnancies go to term, malpresentations such as breech and transverse lie are more frequent. Also, prolonged labor (which is probably due to inadequate muscle development in the uterus), increased bleeding, and a higher incidence of fetal anomalies caused by defective implantation of the placenta all occur more commonly than in normal pregnancies. An intravenous pyelogram or urinary tract ultrasound is mandatory in these patients with müllerian anomalies since there is an associated higher incidence of congenital urinary tract anomalies; approximately 30% of patients with müllerian anomalies have coexisting urinary tract anomalies. In bicornuate uterus (termed uterus bicornis unicollis), there is a double uterine cavity (bicornis) and a single cervix (unicollis) with a normal vagina.

286–290. The answers are 286-d, 287-b, 288-a, 289-a, 290-c. _(Ransom 1997, pp 271–275.)_ True sexual precocity in girls is characterized by normal gonadotropin levels (as opposed to expected low prepubertal gonadotropin levels) and a normal ovulatory pattern. It represents premature activation of a normally operating hypothalamic-pituitary axis. Although it is usually idiopathic, true sexual precocity can arise from cerebral causes such as tumors or a history of encephalitis or meningitis, as well as from hypothyroidism, polyostotic fibrous dysplasia, neurofibromatosis, and other disorders. In girls who have precocious pseudopuberty, the endocrine glands, usually under neoplastic influences, produce elevated amounts of estrogens (isosexual precocious pseudopuberty) or androgens (heterosexual precocious pseudopuberty). Ovarian tumors appear to be the most common cause of isosexual precocious pseudopuberty; some ovarian tumors, including dysgerminomas and choriocarcinomas, can produce so much gonadotropin that pregnancy tests are positive. Incomplete sexual precocity, which is usually idiopathic, is characterized by only partial sexual maturity, such as premature thelarche or premature adrenarche (pubarche). Incomplete sexual precocity can be accompanied by abnormal function of the central nervous system (e.g., mental deficiency). Gonadotropin levels are frequently normal in these patients. In gonadotropin-producing tumors, high levels of gonadotropins such as FSH are produced with subsequent production of estrogen. Examples of these rare tumors are hepatoma, chorioepithelioma, and presacral tumors.

291–295. The answers are 291-d, 292-a, 293-b, 294-e, 295-c. (*Rock, 8/e, pp 63–94.*) The blood supply of the pelvic organs and musculature is derived primarily from the hypogastric (internal iliac) artery, which in turn arises from the division of the common iliac into the internal and the external iliac arteries. The uterine artery arises from the anterior division of the hypogastric artery; it supplies the upper vagina, uterus, and fallopian tubes. The bladder is also supplied by the vesical branches of the hypogastric artery, which terminates as the internal pudendal artery, supplying the perineum, labia, and clitoris as well as the thigh muscles. The uterine veins, which drain into the internal iliac veins, generally follow the course of the uterine arteries. Together, the uterine artery and vein course superiorly (i.e., above) to the ureters along the base of the broad ligaments. The two ovarian veins follow different courses. The right ovarian vein drains into the inferior vena cava just below the level of the right renal vein, while the left ovarian vein drains into the left renal vein. The right ovarian vein may become distended during pregnancy, causing partial obstruction of the ureter proximal to its course. This has been postulated to be a cause of right hydronephrosis in pregnancy. The ovarian arteries arise from the abdominal aorta. They course through the infundibulopelvic ligament and supply the ovary and the fallopian tube.

A thorough understanding of these relationships is essential in gynecologic surgery, especially in cases of hemorrhage that require ligation of the hypogastric artery. For example, a ligature placed on the hypogastric artery for control of hemorrhage must be positioned after the origin of the posterior division of the hypogastric artery; this vessel provides parietal branches to the sacrum and gluteal muscles, and ligation would be unnecessary and might cause sloughing of these muscles. Also, the relationship between the uterine arteries and ureters is important; use the phrase "water under the bridge" to help you remember that the ureters pass *under* the uterine blood vessels, an important anatomic relationship during hysterectomy.

SEXUALITY, CONTRACEPTION, ABORTION, AND STERILIZATION

Questions

DIRECTIONS: Each item below contains a question or incomplete statement followed by suggested responses. Select the **one best** response to each question.

296. Which of the following is an undesirable side effect of prostaglandin-induced abortions?

a. Hyperosmolar crisis
b. Birth of a live fetus
c. Water intoxication
d. Rupture of the uterus
e. Peritonitis

297. Which of the following are techniques used for second-trimester abortions?

a. Hysterectomy
b. Prostaglandin E$_2$ vaginal suppositories
c. Intraamniotic oxytocin
d. Suction curettage
e. Administration of RU-486

298. In the experience of Masters and Johnson and other sex therapists, which type of male or female sexual dysfunction has the lowest cure rate?

a. Premature ejaculation
b. Vaginismus
c. Primary impotence
d. Secondary impotence
e. Female orgasmic dysfunction

299. The most common form of contraception used by couples in the United States is

a. Pills
b. Condom
c. Diaphragm
d. Intrauterine device (IUD)
e. Permanent sterilization

300. Which of the following neoplasms has been associated with the use of oral contraceptives?

a. Breast cancer
b. Ovarian cancer
c. Endometrial cancer
d. Hepatic cancer
e. Hepatic adenoma

301. Which of the following is the best explanation for the mechanism of the action of the intrauterine device (IUD)?

a. Hyperperistalsis of the fallopian tubes accelerates oocyte transport and prevents fertilization
b. A subacute or chronic bacterial endometritis interferes with implantation
c. Premature endometrial sloughing associated with menorrhagia causes early abortion
d. A sterile inflammatory response of the endometrium prevents implantation
e. Cervical mucus is rendered impenetrable to migrating sperm

302. The major cause of unplanned pregnancies in women using oral contraceptives is

a. Breakthrough ovulation at midcycle
b. A high frequency of intercourse
c. Incorrect use of oral contraceptives
d. Gastrointestinal malabsorption
e. Development of antibodies

303. An intrauterine pregnancy of approximately 10 wk gestation is confirmed in a 30-year-old gravida 5, para 4 woman with an IUD in place. The patient expresses a strong desire for the pregnancy to be continued. On examination the string of the IUD is noted to be protruding from the cervical os. The most appropriate course of action is to

a. Leave the IUD in place without any other treatment
b. Leave the IUD in place and continue prophylactic antibiotics throughout pregnancy
c. Remove the IUD immediately
d. Terminate the pregnancy because of the high risk of infection
e. Perform a laparoscopy to rule out a heterotopic ectopic pregnancy

304. Which of the following statements is true regarding spermicides found in vaginal foams, creams, and suppositories?

a. The active agent in these spermicides is nonoxynol-9
b. The active agent in these spermicides is levonorgestrel
c. Effectiveness is higher in younger users
d. Effectiveness is higher than that of the diaphragm
e. These agents are associated with an increased incidence of congenital malformations

305. According to Masters and Johnson, which of the following factors increase the likelihood of female orgasm during sexual intercourse?

a. A larger clitoral glans
b. A clitoris located closer to the vaginal introitus
c. Erection of the clitoral shaft
d. Male superior coital position
e. Traction on the clitoral hood by the labia minora

306. Which of the following is a true statement regarding primary orgasmic dysfunction in women?

a. It is unrelated to partner behavior
b. The influence of orthodox religious beliefs is still of major etiologic significance
c. It is unrelated to partner sexual performance
d. It is not associated with a history of rape
e. A woman affected by it has had an orgasm with another partner

307. The plateau phase of sexual excitement in women includes which of the following physiologic responses?

a. Areolar detumescence
b. Decreased systolic blood pressure
c. Involuntary contractions of the rectal sphincter
d. Skeletal muscle relaxation
e. Deep vasocongestion

308. A 19-year-old woman presents for voluntary termination of pregnancy 6 wk after her expected (missed) menses. She previously had regular menses every 28 days. Pregnancy is confirmed by β-human chorionic gonadotropin (β-hCG) and ultrasound confirms expected gestational age. Which technique for termination of pregnancy would be safe and effective in this patient at this time?

a. Dilatation and evacuation (D&E)
b. Hypertonic saline infusion
c. Suction dilatation and curettage (D&C)
d. 15-methyl α-prostaglandin injection
e. Hysterotomy

309. Components of the natural lubrication produced by the female during sexual arousal and intercourse include which of the following?

a. Fluid from Skene's glands
b. Mucus produced by endocervical glands
c. Viscous fluid from Bartholin's glands
d. Transudate-like material from the vaginal walls
e. Uterotubal fluid

310. A 62-year-old woman presents for annual examination. Her last spontaneous menstrual period was 9 years ago, and she has been reluctant to use postmenopausal hormone replacement because of a strong family history of breast cancer. She now complains of diminished interest in sexual activity. Which of the following is the most likely cause of her complaint?

a. Decreased vaginal length
b. Decreased ovarian function
c. Alienation from her partner
d. Untreatable sexual dysfunction
e. Physiologic anorgasmia

311. A 22-year-old nulliparous woman has recently become sexually active. She consults you because of painful coitus, with the pain located at the vaginal introitus. It is accompanied by painful involuntary contraction of the pelvic muscles. Other than confirmation of these findings, the pelvic examination is normal. Of the following, what is the most common cause of this condition?

a. Endometriosis
b. Psychogenic causes
c. Bartholin's gland abscess
d. Vulvar atrophy
e. Ovarian cyst

312. A 39-year-old patient is contemplating discontinuing birth control pills in order to conceive. She is concerned about her fertility at this age, and inquires about when she can anticipate resumption of normal menses. You counsel her that by 3 mo after discontinuation of birth control pills, the following proportion of patients will resume normal menses

a. 99%
b. 95%
c. 80%
d. 50%
e. 5%

313. Which of the following is an absolute contraindication to the use of combination oral contraceptive pills?

a. Varicose veins
b. Tension headache
c. Seizure disorders
d. Obesity and smoking in women over 35 years of age
e. Mild essential hypertension

314. You are evaluating the laboratory results of a patient on oral contraceptive pills. Use of the birth control pill decreases which of the following?

a. Glucose tolerance
b. Binding globulins
c. High-density lipoprotein (HDL) cholesterol
d. Triglycerides
e. Hemoglobin concentration

315. In combination birth control pills, the contraceptive effect of the estrogenic component is primarily related to

a. Conversion of ethinyl estradiol to mestranol
b. Atrophy of the endometrium
c. Suppression of cervical mucus secretion
d. Suppression of luteinizing hormone (LH) secretion
e. Suppression of follicle-stimulating hormone (FSH) secretion

316. Which of the following mechanisms best explains the contraceptive effect of birth control pills that contain both synthetic estrogen and progestin?

a. Direct inhibition of oocyte maturation
b. Inhibition of ovulation
c. Production of uterine secretions that are toxic to developing embryos
d. Impairment of implantation hyperplastic changes of the endometrium
e. Impairment of sperm transport due to uterotubal obstruction

317. Five patients present for contraceptive counseling, each requesting that an IUD be inserted. A prior history of which of the following is a recognized contraindication to the insertion of an IUD?

a. Pelvic inflammatory disease
b. Pregnancy with an IUD
c. Dysfunctional uterine bleeding
d. Cervicitis
e. Chorioamnionitis

318. In addition to effective contraception, health benefits for women taking oral contraceptives include a decreased incidence of which of the following?

a. Lung cancer
b. Benign breast disease
c. Hypertension
d. Cervical cancer
e. Pelvic inflammatory disease

319. True statements regarding operative procedures for sterilization include which of the following?

a. They cannot be performed immediately postpartum
b. They have become the second most common method of contraception for white couples between 20 and 40 years of age in the United States
c. They can be considered effective immediately in females (bilateral tubal ligation)
d. They can be considered effective immediately in males (vasectomy)
e. Tubal ligation should be performed in the secretory phase of the menstrual cycle

320. A 34-year-old male undergoes vasectomy. Which of the following is the most frequent immediate complication of this procedure?

a. Infection
b. Impotence
c. Hematoma
d. Spontaneous reanastomosis
e. Sperm granulomas

DIRECTIONS: Each group of questions below consists of lettered options followed by numbered items. For each numbered item, select the appropriate lettered option(s). Each lettered option may be used once, more than once, or not at all. **Choose exactly the number of options indicated following each item.**

Items 321–325

For each female patient below seeking contraception, select the method that is medically contraindicated for that patient.

a. Oral contraceptives
b. IUD
c. Condoms
d. Laparoscopic tubal ligation
e. Diaphragm

321. A woman with multiple sexual partners **(SELECT 1 METHOD)**

322. A woman with a history of deep vein thrombosis **(SELECT 1 METHOD)**

323. A woman with moderate cystocele **(SELECT 1 METHOD)**

324. A woman with severely reduced functional capacity as a result of chronic obstructive lung disease **(SELECT 1 METHOD)**

325. A woman with a known latex allergy **(SELECT 1 METHOD)**

Items 326–332

For the following methods of contraception, select the most appropriate rate of use effectiveness (failure rate or percentage of pregnancies per year of actual patient use).

a. 80%
b. 40%
c. 15% to 25%
d. 5% to 15%
e. 3% to 10%

326. Rhythm method **(SELECT 1 RATE)**

327. IUD **(SELECT 1 RATE)**

328. Diaphragm **(SELECT 1 RATE)**

329. Postcoital douche **(SELECT 1 RATE)**

330. Oral contraceptive **(SELECT 1 RATE)**

331. Condom and spermicidal agent **(SELECT 1 RATE)**

332. Condom alone **(SELECT 1 RATE)**

Items 333–338

For each situation listed below involving oral contraceptives, select the most appropriate response.

a. Stop pills and resume after 7 days
b. Continue pills as usual
c. Continue pills and use an additional form of contraception
d. Take an additional pill
e. Stop pills and seek a medical examination

333. Nausea during first cycle of pills **(SELECT 1 RESPONSE)**

334. No menses during 7 days following 21-day cycle of correct use **(SELECT 1 RESPONSE)**

335. Pill forgotten for 1 day **(SELECT 1 RESPONSE)**

336. Pill forgotten for 10 continuous days **(SELECT 1 RESPONSE)**

337. Light bleeding at midcycle during 1st mo on pill **(SELECT 1 RESPONSE)**

338. Hemoptysis **(SELECT 1 RESPONSE)**

SEXUALITY, CONTRACEPTION, ABORTION, AND STERILIZATION

Answers

296. The answer is b. (*Mishell, 3/e, pp 341–344. Rock, 8/e, pp 491–492. James, 2/e, pp 1079–1090.*) An occasional troublesome feature of prostaglandin-induced abortions is the expulsion of a fetus with signs of life. Hyperosmolar crisis and peritonitis are specific complications following intraamniotic injection of hypertonic saline, a procedure no longer generally used. Water intoxication can be seen following administration of both saline (which is outmoded) and intravenous oxytocin. Rupture of the uterus has been documented from oxytocin infused after intraamniotic prostaglandin F2$_\alpha$ and, rarely, from oxytocin given during the first half of pregnancy in women of high parity.

297. The answer is b. (*Mishell, 3/e, pp 341–344. Rock, 8/e, pp 491–492. James, 2/e, pp 1079–1090.*) None of the methods listed in the question are used for second-trimester terminations except prostaglandin E$_2$ vaginal suppositories. Induction of labor with intravenous (never intraamniotic) oxytocin in the second trimester requires very large doses with concomitant risks of water intoxication from antidiuretic hormone activity; however, oxytocin can be used intravenously to augment contractions once labor has been initiated. Intraamniotic prostaglandin F$_{2\alpha}$ and intramuscularly injected 15-methyl α-prostaglandin are both effective for induction of labor. The antiprostaglandin RU-486 is used for the voluntary termination of early (first-trimester) pregnancy; however, it is not approved for this indication in the United States. Hysterectomy is not indicated for termination of pregnancy unless there is a life-threatening maternal condition for which hysterectomy is otherwise indicated.

298. The answer is c. (*Mishell, 3/e, pp 171, 181–182.*) In a 5-year follow-up study of couples treated by Masters and Johnson, the cure rates for vaginismus and premature ejaculation approached 100%. Orgasmic dysfunction was corrected in 80% of women, and secondary impotence (impotence despite a history of previous coital success) resolved in 70% of men. Primary impotence (chronic and complete inability to maintain an erection sufficient for coitus) had the worst prognosis, with cure reported in only approximately 50% of cases. Other therapists report very similar statistics.

299. The answer is e. (*Mishell, 3/e, pp 284–285.*) In studies of contraceptive methods used by reproductive age women in the United States, 31.9% used permanent sterilization (tubal ligation by any method for themselves or vasectomy for their partners). Oral contraception was used by 27.4% of women exposed, and barrier methods of contraception were used by 17.5% of women surveyed.

300. The answer is e. (*Mishell, 3/e, pp 321–323.*) Beginning with high-dose combination contraceptive pills used over 20 years ago, pills have been studied extensively for a possible association with neoplasia. There is only scant evidence from this more than 20 years of experience that use of oral contraceptives increases the risk of any type of cancer. Actually, the progestational component of combination pills (or progestin-only mini-pills) may confer a protective effect against carcinoma of the breast and endometrium, and avoiding ovulation may decrease the risk of developing ovarian carcinoma. A slightly higher risk of cervical carcinoma was observed in some studies of users of oral contraceptives. These studies were not controlled, however, for confounding variables such as multiple partners or age at onset of sexual intercourse, and it is generally believed now that any increased risk in contraceptive pill users would be attributable to these other factors and not the steroids themselves. Although the risk of developing benign liver adenomas is increased somewhat in users of oral contraceptives, the risk of hepatic carcinoma is not increased.

301. The answer is d. (*Speroff, 6/e, p 980.*) It is currently believed that alteration in the cellular and biochemical components of the endometrium occurs with the IUD, culminating in the development of a sterile inflammatory reaction. Polymorphonuclear leukocytes, giant cells, plasma cells, and macrophages are seen in the endometrium after placement. Biochemical changes in the endometrium include changing levels of lysosomal hydrolases, glycogen deposition, oxygen composition, total proteins, acid and alkaline phosphatases, urea phospholipids, and RNA/DNA ratios. IUDs treated with copper and progesterone exert additional effects. In sum, these cellular and biochemical effects result in an endometrium that is not conducive to implantation. No effects on the fallopian tubes or systemic hormone levels have been identified, nor is a bacterial endometritis produced.

302. The answer is c. *(Speroff, 6/e, p 925.)* The pregnancy rate with birth control pills, based on theoretical effectiveness, is 0.1%. However, the pregnancy rate in actual use is 0.7%. This increase is due to incorrect use of the pills. Breakthrough ovulation on combination birth control pills, when the pills are taken correctly, is thought to be a very rare occurrence. Unintended pregnancy in women correctly using oral contraceptive pills is not related to sexual frequency, gastrointestinal disturbances, or the development of antibodies.

303. The answer is c. *(Mishell, 3/e, pp 330–339.)* Although there is an increased risk of spontaneous abortion, and a small risk of infection, an intrauterine pregnancy can occur and continue successfully to term with an IUD in place. However, if the patient wishes to keep the pregnancy and if the string is visible, the IUD should be removed in an attempt to reduce the risk of infection, abortion, or both. Although the incidence of ectopic pregnancies with an IUD was at one time thought to be increased, it is now recognized that in fact the overall incidence is unchanged. The apparent increase is the result of the dramatic decrease in intrauterine implantation without affecting ectopic implantation. Thus, while the overall probability of pregnancy is dramatically decreased, when a pregnancy does occur with an IUD in place there is a higher probability that it will be an ectopic one. With this in mind, in the absence of signs and symptoms suggestive of an ectopic pregnancy, especially after ultrasound documentation of an intrauterine pregnancy, laparoscopy is not indicated. The incidence of heterotopic pregnancy, in which intrauterine and extrauterine implantation occur, is no higher than approximately 1 in 2500 pregnancies.

304. The answer is a. *(Mishell, 3/e, p 288. Ransom 1997, p 95. Ransom 2000, p 12.)* All spermicides contain an ingredient, usually nonoxynol-9, that immobilizes or kills sperm on contact. Spermicides provide a mechanical barrier and need to be placed into the vagina before each coital act. Their effectiveness increases with increasing age of the women who use them, probably due to increased motivation. The effectiveness of spermacides is similar to that of the diaphragm, and increases with the concomitant use of condoms. Although it has been reported that contraceptive failures with spermicides may be associated with an increased incidence of congenital malformations, this finding has not been confirmed in several large studies and is not believed to be valid. Levonorgestrel is a synthetic progestational agent found in several combination oral contraceptive pills.

305. The answer is e. *(Mishell, 3/e, pp 179–181.)* Masters and Johnson have shown that the size of the clitoris bears no relation to increased orgasmic capacity. Similarly, the distance between the clitoris and the vaginal introitus makes little difference, because clitoral stimulation during coitus is provided largely by traction on the clitoral hood via the labia minora, which are moved during penile thrusting. Direct clitoral stimulation is achieved by the lateral and female superior coital positions. Erection of the clitoris is likewise not related to orgasmic capacity.

306. The answer is b. *(Mishell, 3/e, pp 179–182.)* Many factors can contribute to the development of primary orgasmic dysfunction in women. By definition, these women will not have been able to achieve orgasm through any means at any time in their lives; reasons for their dysfunction can include the influence of orthodox religious or rigid familial beliefs, dissatisfaction with their partners' behavioral or social traits, or past trauma such as rape. Sexual dysfunction, particularly premature ejaculation in a male partner, can reinforce a woman's orgasmic dysfunction.

307. The answer is e. *(Mishell, 3/e, pp 179–182.)* The response of women to sexual stimulation is generalized and affects many different organ systems. Physiologic responses include superficial and deep vasocongestion accounting for, among other things, enlargement and changes of color of extragenital (including the areolae) and genital areas, as well as systemic blood pressure elevations. Generalized and specific voluntary and involuntary myotonia also may occur, although involuntary contractions of the rectal sphincter are usually detected only during the orgasmic phase of the sexual response.

308. The answer is c. *(Rock, 8/e, pp 485–497.)* Surgical abortion is among the safest procedures in medicine, with a serious complication rate in the first trimester of less than 1% and a mortality of only ½₀ that of term delivery. In the first trimester, suction dilation and curettage is the method of choice. The oral agent RU-486 followed by injection of prostaglandin has been shown to be highly effective and safe in European trials, but as of 2000 this medication was not yet available for clinical use in the United States. It is effective up to about 9 wk of gestation. 15-methyl α-prostaglandin can be used as an intramuscular abortifacient, as can prostaglandin E_2 suppositories or intraamniotic prostaglandin $F2_\alpha$ for second-trimester induction of preterm labor. Intraamniotic injection of hypertonic saline is no longer considered appropriate because it has a much higher incidence of serious complications including death, hyperosmolar crisis, cardiac failure, peritonitis, hemorrhage, and coagulation abnormalities. There are far better medicines available, and saline should no longer be used. Dilatation and evacuation (D&E) is a surgical procedure similar in concept to a dilation and curettage (D&C). However, instead of curettage (scraping) to remove the products of conception, various forceps are placed into the uterine cavity to remove the products of conception. D&E is performed for termination of later pregnancies, generally those in the second trimester. Hysterotomy is a surgical procedure in which the uterus is opened transabdominally and the contents evacuated. It is a procedure done for termination of more advanced pregnancies when all other methods of termination are unsuccessful or contraindicated, or, for example, when retained products of conception cannot be expelled with medication or other mechanical means such as D&E.

309. The answer is d. *(Mishell, 3/e, pp 179–182.)* Masters and Johnson observed a transudate-like fluid emanating from the vaginal walls during sexual response. This mucoid material, which is sufficient for complete vaginal lubrication, is produced by transudation from the venous plexus surrounding the vagina and appears seconds after the initiation of sexual excitement. No activity by Skene's glands was noted, and production of cervical mucus during sexual stimulation was observed in only a few subjects. Fluid from Bartholin's glands appears long after vaginal lubrication is well established; in addition, it appears to make only a minor contribution to lubrication in the late plateau phase. Uterine and tubal secretions do not contribute to this lubrication.

310. The answer is b. (*Lobo, 2/e, pp 438–443.*) Sexuality continues despite aging. However, there are physiologic changes that must be recognized. Diminished ovarian function may lower libido, but estrogen replacement therapy (ERT) may help. Sexual dysfunction can be physiologic, e.g., from lowered libido. As with younger patients, however, lowered libido is in most cases treatable. Because aging does not alter the capacity for orgasm or produce vaginismus, a further evaluation should be initiated if these symptoms persist after a postmenopausal woman is placed on ERT.

311. The answer is b. (*Mishell, 3/e, pp 179–182.*) This patient presents with vaginismus, defined as involuntary painful spasm of the pelvic muscles and vaginal outlet. It is usually psychogenic. It should be differentiated from frigidity, which implies lack of sexual desire, and dyspareunia, which is defined as pelvic and/or back pain or other discomfort associated with sexual activity. This pain may be psychogenic in origin, or may be caused by pelvic pathology such as adhesions, endometriosis, or leiomyomas. Treatment of vaginismus is primarily psychotherapeutic as organic vulvar (such as atrophy, Bartholin's gland cyst, or abscess) or pelvic causes are very rare. Vaginismus should be differentiated from dyspareunia, which is deep pelvic pain with coitus; dyspareunia is frequently associated with pelvic pathology such as endometriosis, pelvic adhesions, or ovarian neoplasms.

312. The answer is c. (*Mishell, 3/e, pp 1054–1055.*) Though the estimated incidence of postpill amenorrhea is given as 0.7% to 0.8%, there is no evidence to support the idea that oral contraception causes amenorrhea. Eighty percent of women resume normal periods within 3 mo of ceasing use of the pill, and 95% to 98% resume normal ovulation within 1 year. If there were a true relationship between the pill and amenorrhea, one would expect an increase in infertility in the pill-using population. This has not been found. Infertility rates are the same for those who have used the pill and those who have not. Patients who have not resumed normal periods 12 mo after stopping use of the pill should be evaluated as any other patient with secondary amenorrhea. Women who have irregular menstrual periods are more likely to develop secondary amenorrhea whether they take the pill or not.

313. The answer is d. (*Mishell, 3/e, pp 312–313.*) Absolute contraindications to the use of birth control pills include (1) thromboembolic disorders [deep venous thrombosis (DVT), cerebrovascular accident (CVA), myocardial infarction (MI), or conditions predisposing to these conditions]; (2) markedly impaired liver function; (3) known or suspected carcinoma of the breast or other estrogen-dependent malignancies; (4) undiagnosed abnormal genital malignancies; (5) undiagnosed abnormal genital bleeding; (6) known or suspected bleeding; (7) known or suspected pregnancy; (8) a history of obstructive jaundice in pregnancy; (9) congenital hyperlipidemia; and (10) obesity in women who are smokers and over age 35. Relative contraindications to the use of the birth control pill require clinical judgment and informed consent. These include (1) migraine headaches; (2) hypertension; (3) uterine leiomyomas; (4) gestational diabetes; (5) elective surgery; and (6) seizure disorders.

314. The answer is a. (*Mishell, 3/e, pp 302–313.*) Combination-type oral contraceptives are potent systemic steroids that may cause many detectable alterations in metabolic function, such as increases in binding globulins, bromsulphalein retention, triglycerides and total phospholipids, and a decrease in glucose tolerance. Thus, the benefits of birth control pills must be weighed carefully against the added risks in patients with diabetes, cardiovascular disease, or liver disease. The pill modestly increases HDL cholesterol levels, but should have no direct effect on hemoglobin concentration. In fact, since bleeding volume is generally diminished in birth control pill users, hemoglobin concentration often increases in these patients.

315. The answer is e. (*Mishell, 3/e, pp 291–295.*) The two estrogenic compounds used in oral contraceptives are ethinyl estradiol and its 3-methyl ether, mestranol. To become biologically effective, mestranol must be demethylated to ethinyl estradiol, because mestranol does not bind to the estrogenic cytosol receptor. The degree of conversion of mestranol to ethinyl estradiol varies among individuals; however, it is estimated that ethinyl estradiol is about 1.7 times as potent as the same weight of mestranol. The estrogenic component of birth control pills was originally added to control irregular endometrial desquamation resulting in undesirable vaginal bleeding. However, these estrogens imposed possible risks that would not be inherent in the progestational component alone. For example, thrombosis, the most serious side effect of the pill, is directly related to the dose of estrogen. The higher the estrogen dose, the more likely there will be thrombotic complications.

The combination pill prevents ovulation by inhibiting gonadotropin secretion and exerting its principal effect on pituitary and hypothalamic centers. Progesterone primarily suppresses LH secretion, while estrogen primarily suppresses FSH secretion. The progestational effect of the pill will always take precedence over the estrogenic effect unless the estrogen dose is dramatically increased. Progestogens are responsible for endometrial changes that result in an environment not conducive to implantation, and production of cervical mucus that retards sperm migration.

316. The answer is b. *(Speroff, 6/e, p 879.)* The marked effectiveness of the combined oral contraceptive pill, which contains a synthetic estrogen and a progestin, is related to its multiple antifertility actions. The primary effect is to suppress gonadotropins at the time of the midcycle LH surge, thus inhibiting ovulation. The prolonged progestational effect also causes thickening of the cervical mucus and atrophic (not hyperplasic) changes of the endometrium, thus impairing sperm penetrability and ovum implantation, respectively. Progestational agents in oral contraceptives work by a negative feedback mechanism to inhibit the secretion of LH and, as a result, prevent ovulation. They also cause decidualization and atrophy of the endometrium, hence making implantation impossible. In addition, cervical mucus, which at ovulation is thin and watery, is changed by the influence of progestational agents to a tenacious compound that severely limits sperm motility. Some evidence indicates that progestational agents may change ovum and sperm migration patterns within the reproductive system. Progestins do not prevent irregular bleeding. Estrogen in birth control pills enhances the negative feedback of the progestins and stabilizes the endometrium to prevent irregular menses. Oral contraceptives have no direct effect on oocyte maturation, and do not cause uterotubal obstruction.

317. The answer is a. *(Mishell, 3/e, pp 338–339.)* A previous pregnancy with an IUD is not a contraindication to the use of an IUD. The risk of another pregnancy with the IUD in place is not increased. Previous cervical surgery in the face of a normal Pap smear and no cervical stenosis is not a contraindication to IUD use. The Food and Drug Administration (FDA) lists the following contraindications to the use of an IUD: (1) pregnancy; (2) pelvic inflammatory disease—acute, chronic, or recurrent; (3) acute cervicitis; (4) postpartum endometritis or septic abortion; (5) undiagnosed genital bleeding; (6) gynecologic malignancy; (7) congenital anomalies or uterine fibroids that distort the uterine cavity; and (8) copper allergy (for IUDs that contain copper). Other conditions that might preclude IUD insertion include (1) previous ectopic pregnancy; (2) severe cervical stenosis; (3) severe dysmenorrhea; (4) menometrorrhagia; (5) coagulopathies; and (6) congenital or valvular heart disease.

318. The answer is b. (*Speroff, 6/e, pp 922–925.*) Oral contraceptives offer many noncontraceptive health benefits. Women who are using combination oral contraceptives are less likely to develop cancer of the endometrium than women who do not use oral contraceptives, probably because the formulations contain a progestogen as well as an estrogen. Since progestogens counteract the stimulatory action of the estrogen on target tissues, women who take oral contraceptives rarely have endometrial hyperplasia and appear to have a lower incidence of nonmalignant cystic disease of the breast. Secondary to the antiestrogenic action of progestin, there is a reduction in the amount of blood loss at the time of endometrial shedding; thus, the development of iron-deficiency anemia is less likely. Users of oral contraceptives are at higher risk for cervical neoplasia, and they definitely require annual screening; however, there is no evidence that the oral contraceptives are the causative factor in this increased risk. A more likely explanation is the presence of confounding factors in contraceptive users that increase the risk, such as multiple sexual partners or regular coitus beginning at an earlier age.

319. The answer is c. (*Speroff, 6/e, pp 840–854.*) Sterilization has become the most commonly used method of contraception in the United States. In an otherwise uncomplicated pregnancy, a tubal ligation can, if desired, be performed in the immediate postpartum period. Unless the woman has already conceived at the time of the procedure (which is why tubal ligation should generally be performed in the first half of the cycle, the proliferative phase), the contraceptive effect is immediate. Vasectomy in the male, however, should not be considered effective until an examination of the ejaculate is sperm-free on two successive occasions. Tubal ligation can be performed at any time of the ovarian or endometrial cycle, without regard to endometrial development. Most practitioners prefer to perform tubal ligation right after completion of menses (ie., prior to ovulation) only to obviate the concern that a fertilized oocyte or early embryo could have already passed the ligation area and migrated into the uterus, thus resulting in a pregnancy implanting in the same cycle that the fallopian tubes are ligated.

320. The answer is c. *(Mishell, 3/e, pp 339–340.)* Vasectomy is performed by isolating the vas deferens, cutting it, and closing the ends by either fulguration or ligation. Complications that may arise include hematoma in up to 5% of subjects, sperm granulomas (inflammatory responses to sperm leakage), spontaneous reanastomosis, and, rarely, infections. Sexual function following healing is rarely affected.

321–325. The answers are 321-b, 322-a, 323-e, 324-d, 325-c. *(Mishell, 3/e, pp 283–300.)* Oral contraceptives are the contraceptive method of choice in the motivated, healthy, monogamous young woman. If the pill is properly used, the failure rate for users is the lowest among women using a reversible method of contraception. However, the use of oral contraceptives is contraindicated in patients with a history of thrombophlebitis. Both condoms and the diaphragm, used in conjunction with spermicides, are effective contraceptives that are also effective in preventing sexually transmitted diseases and acquired immune deficiency syndrome (AIDS). The diaphragm should, however, carefully fit in the vagina and is not applicable, therefore, to women with anatomic distortion of the vagina. Latex condoms should not be used in women with a known latex allergy. IUDs are associated with increased risk of salpingitis and ectopic pregnancy, and therefore should be avoided in patients with a history of pelvic inflammatory disease (PID), multiple sexual partners, or ectopic conception. Although tubal ligation may be considered in the patient with chronic obstructive lung disease, the risk of general anesthesia and surgical intervention in this patient is probably high enough to indicate a more conservative approach, such as the use of an IUD.

326–332. The answers are 326-b, 327-e, 328-c, 329-a, 330-d, 331-d, 332-c. *(Mishell, 3/e, pp 283–288.)* There are two methods of describing the effectiveness of contraceptive agents: the theoretical or method effectiveness rate and the actual use effectiveness rate. When comparing different methods, it is important to use comparable figures. The effectiveness of the rhythm method is influenced by the woman's ability to predict the time of ovulation from the regularity of her menses. It is also influenced by the woman's motivation to successfully abstain from intercourse during the 10 days around suspected ovulation. The menstrual and ovulatory irregularities and lapses in the woman's motivation account for a pregnancy rate of 40 with the rhythm method. In contrast to the rhythm method, the IUD requires little or no action on the part of the woman. For this reason the device's actual use effectiveness approaches its maximal theoretical effectiveness, with a pregnancy rate of 3 to 10. Unrecognized expulsion or misplaced insertion of the IUD are responsible for most failures. The vaginal diaphragm and the condom are barrier contraceptives in that for each act of sexual intercourse they pose a barrier between the sperm ejaculate and the endocervical canal. In theory, both can be very effective. However, both require recurrent motivation for application with each act of intercourse. Lapses in motivation are not uncommon, and there is a pregnancy rate of 15 to 25 for each of these two methods. The condom used with a spermicidal agent is very effective, more so than either used alone. The pregnancy rate with postcoital douching is almost the same as that for unprotected intercourse (80). This lack of effectiveness is readily explained by the extremely rapid progression of motile sperm into the endocervical canal. Within several minutes of coitus, sperm have ascended the female reproductive tract and can be found within the endocervical mucus, uterus, and fallopian tubes. Coupled with the failure of a vaginal douche to reach the endocervix, this method is essentially useless. Combined oral contraceptive birth control pills are clearly the most effective reversible contraceptive currently available. With correct use, many studies report a contraceptive effectiveness that approaches 100% (pregnancy rate less than 0.1). This extreme effectiveness is best explained by the pill's multiplicity of actions, i.e., suppression of ovulation, hostility of cervical mucus to sperm penetration, and hostility of atrophic endometrium to the implantation of a conceptus. Failure to take the pills with regularity is responsible for most failures, and in practice pregnancy rates of at least 5% are common.

333–338.   The answers are 333-b, 334-b, 335-d, 336-c, 337-b, 338-e. (Mishell, 3/e, pp 1031–1032, 1039.) Common side effects of birth control pills include nausea, breakthrough bleeding, bloating, and leg cramps. If these side effects are experienced in the first two or three cycles of pills, when they are most common, the pills may be safely continued, as these effects usually remit spontaneously. On occasion, following correct use of a full cycle of pills, withdrawal bleeding may fail to occur (silent menses).

Pregnancy is a very unlikely explanation for this event; therefore, pills should be resumed as usual (after 7 days) just as if bleeding had occurred. However, if a second consecutive period has been missed, pregnancy should be more seriously considered and ruled out by a pregnancy test, medical examination, or both. Women occasionally forget to take pills; however, when only a single pill has been omitted, it can be taken immediately in addition to the usual pill at the usual time. This single-pill omission is associated with little if any loss in effectiveness. If three or more pills are omitted, the pill should be resumed as usual, but an additional contraceptive method (e.g., condoms) should be used through one full cycle. Although most side effects caused by birth control pills can be considered minor, serious side effects do sometimes occur. A painful, swollen calf may signal thrombophlebitis. Hemoptysis may signal pulmonary embolism. Either of these circumstances should be considered a medical emergency, and immediate medical attention should be sought.

INFECTIONS, UROLOGY, ENDOMETRIOSIS, PELVIC RELAXATION, AND SURGERY

Questions

DIRECTIONS: Each item below contains a question or incomplete statement followed by suggested responses. Select the **one best** response to each question.

339. A patient is undergoing evaluation for urinary leakage. Methylene blue is instilled into the urinary bladder, and the blue color is noted to be saturating the tip of a vaginal tampon. In the United States, the most common cause of this condition is

a. Obstetric injury
b. Abdominal hysterectomy
c. Radiation treatment
d. Radical hysterectomy for cervical cancer
e. Vaginal hysterectomy

340. A 45-year-old morbidly obese patient undergoes abdominal hysterectomy for leiomyomas and menorrhagia. On the third postoperative day, you become concerned that the incision is not healing properly. Copious serosanguineous drainage is noted from the incision. The most likely diagnosis is wound

a. Hematoma
b. Dehiscence
c. Evisceration
d. Seroma
e. Infection

341. A 50-year-old woman complains of leakage of urine. After genuine stress urinary incontinence, the most common cause of this urinary leakage is

a. Detrusor dyssynergia
b. Unstable bladder
c. Unstable urethra
d. Urethral diverticulum
e. Overflow incontinence

342. A 65-year-old woman complains of leakage of urine. The most common cause of this condition in this patient is

a. Anatomic stress urinary incontinence
b. Urethral diverticula
c. Overflow incontinence
d. Unstable bladder
e. Fistula

343. A 59-year-old woman undergoes vaginal hysterectomy and anteroposterior repair for uterine prolapse. Which of the following is a complication of this procedure that often develops within 2 wk of surgery?

a. Dyspareunia
b. Stress urinary incontinence
c. Nonfistulous fecal incontinence
d. Enterocele
e. Vaginal vault prolapse

344. A 53-year-old postmenopausal woman, gravida 3, para 3, presents for evaluation of troublesome urinary leakage of 6 wk duration. Of the following choices, which is the most appropriate first step in this patient's evaluation?

a. Urinalysis and culture
b. Urethral pressure profiles
c. Intravenous pyelogram
d. Cystourethrogram
e. Urethrocystoscopy

345. A patient is diagnosed with acute pelvic inflammatory disease (PID). Tender bilateral, palpable masses in both adnexa are confirmed on ultrasound examination. Which of the following agents would you add to this patient's regimen of penicillin and gentamicin?

a. Erythromycin
b. Amoxicillin
c. Doxycycline
d. Clindamycin
e. Cefaclor

346. Which of the following contraceptives appear to increase the risk for development of pelvic inflammatory disease?

a. Condoms without spermicide
b. Oral contraceptives
c. Intrauterine device
d. Diaphragm
e. Vasectomy

347. At the time of annual examination, a patient expresses concern over exposure to sexually transmitted diseases. During your pelvic examination, a singular, indurated, nontender ulcer is noted on the vulva. Venereal Disease Research Laboratory (VDRL) and fluorescent treponemal antibody (FTA) tests are positive. Without treatment, the next stage of this disease is clinically characterized by

a. Optic nerve atrophy and generalized paresis
b. Tabes dorsalis
c. Gummas
d. Macular rash over the hands and feet
e. Aortic aneurysm

348. A 19-year-old college student is being seen for a primary herpes infection with severe vulvar pain, fever, and malaise. Oral acyclovir has documented efficacy in treating this disease by reducing

a. The number of symptomatic days
b. The number of viral particles that settle in the ventral root ganglia
c. Leukocyte infection by active virus
d. The degree of viremia in the chronic, asymptomatic phase of the infection
e. Host immune defenses that increase symptom severity

349. A 19-year-old patient has biopsy-proven extensive vaginal flat condylomas that have recurred after laser treatment 3 mo ago. At this point, the best therapy is to

a. Repeat laser treatment
b. Apply podophyllum
c. Apply trichloroacetic acid
d. Apply 5% 5-fluorouracil cream
e. Perform cryotherapy

350. False-positive Venereal Disease Research Laboratory (VDRL) tests have been associated with which of the following conditions?

a. Narcotics addiction
b. Pneumococcal pneumonia
c. Young age
d. Diabetes mellitus
e. Condyloma accuminata

351. A 24-year-old patient has returned from a year-long stay in the tropics. Four weeks ago she noted a small vulvar ulceration that spontaneously healed. Now there is painful inguinal adenopathy with malaise and fever. You are considering the diagnosis of lymphogranuloma venereum (LGV). The diagnosis can be established by

a. Staining for Donovan bodies
b. The presence of antibodies to *Chlamydia trachomatis*
c. Positive Frei skin test
d. Culturing *Haemophilus ducreyi*
e. Culturing *Calymmatobacterium granulomatis*

352. A postmenopausal woman is undergoing evaluation for fecal incontinence. She has no other diagnosed medical problems. She lives by herself and is self-sufficient, oriented, and an excellent historian. Physical examination is completely normal. Which of the following is the most likely cause of this patient's condition?

a. Rectal prolapse
b. Diabetes
c. Obstetrical trauma
d. Senility
e. Excessive caffeine intake

353. You are discussing surgical options with a patient with symptomatic pelvic relaxation. Partial colpocleisis (Le Fort procedure) may be more appropriate than vaginal hysterectomy and anterior and posterior (A&P) repair for patients who

a. Do not desire retained sexual function
b. Need periodic endometrial sampling
c. Have had endometrial dysplasia
d. Have cervical dysplasia that requires colposcopic evaluation
e. Have a history of urinary incontinence

354. Which of the following factors is most important in the subsequent development of genital prolapse?

a. Poor tissue quality
b. Chronic straining at bowel movements
c. Menopause
d. Childbirth trauma
e. Multiple deliveries

355. Which of the following predispose to vascular laparoscopic complications?

a. A sharp trocar
b. Tight pneumoperitoneum
c. Insertion of the trocar through a scar
d. Multiparity
e. Acute angular entry of the trocar

356. For the treatment of stress urinary incontinence, you are assisting in a procedure in which the periurethral tissue is attached to the symphysis pubis. The disadvantages of this Marshall-Marchetti-Krantz procedure compared with other surgical alternatives for treatment of stress urinary incontinence include which of the following?

a. Urinary retention
b. Increased incidence of urinary tract infections
c. High failure rate
d. Osteitis pubis

357. Urethral diverticula are most often caused by which of the following?

a. Congenital factors
b. Bacterial infection
c. Urethral stricture
d. Estrogen deprivation
e. Trauma

358. A patient is seen on the second postoperative day after a difficult abdominal hysterectomy complicated by hemorrhage from the left uterine artery pedicle. Multiple sutures were placed into this area to control bleeding. The patient now has fever, left back pain, left costovertebral angle tenderness, and hematuria. An ultrasound examination shows that fluid has accumulated in the left flank. The most likely diagnosis is

a. Postoperative hemorrhage
b. Bowel obstruction
c. Formation of a wound seroma
d. Abscess formation
e. Ureteral injury

359. If the injury in the patient described above had been recognized at the time of surgery, which of the following procedures could have been recommended?

a. Percutaneous nephrostomy
b. Placement of a ureteral stent without anastomosis
c. Intraperitoneal drainage without anastomosis
d. Ureteroureteral anastomosis
e. Ureteral reimplantation into the bladder

360. In a patient who complains of urinary incontinence, a cystometrogram is performed to

a. Determine urethral length
b. Rule out an unstable trigone
c. Diagnose stress urinary incontinence
d. Determine if a patient has normal bladder sensation
e. Diagnose ureterovesical reflux

361. Which of the following primary treatments is most appropriate for this patient with extensive vulvar lesions shown below?

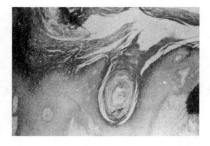

a. Application of podophyllum
b. 5-fluorouracil
c. Morcellation
d. Simple vulvectomy
e. Local excision

362. A patient complains of a recurrent vaginal discharge despite multiple treatment courses. Tests likely to be diagnostic include

a. Fungal culture
b. Bimanual examination
c. KOH suspension for microscopic examination
d. Noting the color of the discharge
e. Serology

363. One day after a casual sexual encounter with a bisexual man recently diagnosed as antibody-positive for human immunodeficiency virus (HIV), a patient is concerned whether she may have become infected. A negative antibody titer is obtained. To test for seroconversion, when is the earliest you should reschedule repeat antibody testing after the sexual encounter?

a. 1 to 2 wk
b. 3 to 4 wk
c. 6 to 12 wk
d. 12 to 15 wk
e. 26 to 52 wk

DIRECTIONS: Each group of questions below consists of lettered options followed by numbered items. For each numbered item, select the appropriate lettered option(s). Each lettered option may be used once, more than once, or not at all. **Choose exactly the number of options indicated following each item.**

Items 364–368

Match the descriptions below with the appropriate infectious agent or condition.

a. *Candida albicans*
b. *Trichomonas vaginalis*
c. *Neisseria gonorrhoeae*
d. *Gardnerella vaginalis* (formerly *Haemophilus vaginalis*)
e. Atrophic (senile) vaginitis

364. A frequent cause of non-specific vaginitis **(SELECT 1 MATCH)**

365. Predisposition for those with diabetes mellitus **(SELECT 1 MATCH)**

366. Causes production of a frothy discharge **(SELECT 1 MATCH)**

367. Causes production of a grossly recognizable vaginal mucosa with punctate hemorrhage ("strawberry spots") **(SELECT 1 MATCH)**

368. Can be effectively treated with an estrogen cream **(SELECT 1 MATCH)**

Items 369–372

For each patient below, select the appropriate antibiotic.

a. Tetracycline
b. Procaine penicillin
c. Metronidazole
d. Benzathine penicillin
e. Spectinomycin

369. A 35-year-old woman recently diagnosed as having primary syphilis. **(SELECT 1 ANTIBIOTIC)**

370. A 23-year-old woman with acute salpingitis who is being treated with gentamicin and clindamycin but not responding. Culture of the cervix is positive for chlamydia. **(SELECT 1 ANTIBIOTIC)**

371. A 34-year-old patient with a tubo-ovarian abscess who was started on penicillin and gentamicin. Purulent material aspirated from the cul-de-sac has revealed *Bacteroides fragilis*. The patient has failed to respond clinically to the two antibiotics given. **(SELECT 1 ANTIBIOTIC)**

372. A 28-year-old woman with a penicillinase-producing *Neisseria gonorrhoeae* **(SELECT 1 ANTIBIOTIC)**

INFECTIONS, UROLOGY, ENDOMETRIOSIS, PELVIC RELAXATION, AND SURGERY

Answers

339. The answer is b. *(Scott, 8/e, pp 763–764.)* The finding of blue dye on the tip of the tampon confirms the presence of either a ureterovaginal or vesicovaginal fistula (or both). In developing countries, obstetric injury remains the leading cause of vesicovaginal fistulas. In this country, vesicovaginal fistulas rarely occur after obstetric deliveries. Although fistulas can occur after radiation treatment, radical hysterectomy, or vaginal hysterectomy, they are three times more common with abdominal hysterectomy. It is thought that inadequate mobilization of the bladder or blunt dissection of the bladder from the pubovesical fascia results in the formation of fistulas. Although simple drainage will cure small fistulas, usually surgical intervention is required to correct the problem.

340. The answer is c. *(Rock, 8/e, pp 310–311.)* Wound dehiscence refers to separation of the incision from the level of the skin to and including the underlying fascia, while evisceration is a wound dehiscence in which peritoneal contents (large or small bowel, omentum) prolapse to the exterior. Serosanguineous drainage occurs very frequently before evisceration from the incision. Drainage can be accompanied by pain or by the feeling that something is "giving way." Prompt surgical repair is mandatory. In patients such as this one in which there is a high risk of wound dehiscence, special suture techniques to strengthen the fascial incision are employed. These include Smead-Jones closure or placement of retention sutures.

341. The answer is b. *(Scott, 8/e, pp 768–770.)* Stress incontinence is the involuntary loss of urine when intravesical pressure exceeds the maximum urethral pressure in the absence of detrusor activity. The most common cause of urinary incontinence is incompetence of the urethral sphincter, termed genuine stress incontinence. The other major cause of incontinence is unstable bladder. An unstable bladder is the occurrence of involuntary, uninhibited detrusor contractions of greater than 15 cm H_2O with simultaneous urethral relaxation. The incidence of patients with incontinence due to an unstable bladder can vary up to approximately 60% of patients presenting with incontinence. Other causes of urinary incontinence are less common and include overflow secondary to urinary retention, congenital abnormalities, infections, fistulas, detrusor dyssynergia, and urethral diverticula. Detrusor dyssynergia implies that when the patient has an uninhibited detrusor contraction, there is simultaneous contraction of the urethral or periurethral striated muscle (normally there is urethral relaxation with a detrusor contraction). This is generally seen in patients with neurologic lesions. Urethral diverticula classically present with dribbling incontinence after voiding.

342. The answer is d. *(Scott, 8/e, pp 767–768.)* As patients age, the incidence of vesicle instability or unstable bladder increases dramatically. Although estrogen has been reported to decrease urgency, frequency, and nocturia in menopausal women, its effect on correction of stress urinary incontinence or vesicle instability is unclear. In the elderly population there are also many transient causes of incontinence that the physician should consider. These include dementia, medications (especially α-adrenergic blockers), decreased patient mobility, endocrine abnormalities (hypercalcemia, hypothyroidism), stool impaction, and urinary tract infections.

343. The answer is b. *(Mishell, 3/e, pp 738–741.)* Many patients who have uterine prolapse or a large protuberant cystocele will be continent because of urethral obstruction caused by the cystocele or prolapse. In fact, at times these patients may need to reduce the prolapse in order to void. Following surgical repair, if the urethrovesical junction is not properly elevated, urinary incontinence may result. This incontinence may present within the first few days following surgery. Dyspareunia can be caused by shortening of the vagina or constriction at the introitus after healing is complete. If the vaginal vault is not properly suspended and the uterosacral ligaments plicated, vaginal vault prolapse or enterocele may occur at a later date. Fecal incontinence is not a complication of vaginal hysterectomy with repair. It may occur, however, if a fistula is formed through unrecognized damage to the rectal mucosa.

344. The answer is a. (*Scott, 8/e, p 753. Rock, 8/e, pp 1088–1089.*) When patients present with urinary incontinence, a urinalysis and culture should be performed. In patients diagnosed with a urinary tract infection, treatment should be initiated and then the patient should be reevaluated. It is not uncommon for symptoms of urinary leakage to resolve after appropriate therapy. After obtaining the history and physical examination and evaluating a urinalysis (including urine culture), initial evaluation of the incontinent patient includes a cystometrogram, check for residual urine volume, stress test, and urinary diary. A cystometrogram is a test that determines urethral and bladder pressures as a function of bladder volume; also noted are the volumes and pressures when the patient first has the sensation of need to void, when maximal bladder capacity is reached, etc. Residual urine volume is determined by bladder catheterization after the patient has voided; when urine remains after voiding, infection and incontinence may result.

345. The answer is d. (*Rock, 8/e, pp 661–664.*) This patient has acute PID (acute salpingitis) with bilateral tubo-ovarian abscesses. Treatment regimens for acute salpingitis with tubo-ovarian abscesses should include agents active against gonorrhea, gram-negative rods (intestinal flora), and anaerobic organisms (e.g., *Bacteroides fragilis*). Doxycycline has been added to many regimens to cover chlamydial infection. There is no single agent active against the entire spectrum of pathogens. The combination of penicillin and gentamicin is inadequate because it fails to cover anaerobic organisms and chlamydia. Agents active against anaerobic organisms include clindamycin and metronidazole.

346. The answer is c. (*Rock, 8/e, pp 661–664.*) Acute salpingitis, or pelvic inflammatory disease (PID), is a disease predominantly of nulliparous young women. The intrauterine device (IUD) increases the risk of developing salpingitis three- to fivefold; the number of sexual partners and the incidence of sexually transmitted disease in a population also influence the development of PID in IUD users. Oral contraceptives are felt to have a protective effect on developing infections; the risk is 30% to 90% that of nonusers. Condoms, diaphragms, and chemical barriers also provide protection from disease. Vasectomy does not appear to influence the risk for development of PID.

347. The answer is d. *(Ransom 1997, p 52.)* Syphilis is a chronic disease produced by the spirochete *Treponema pallidum*. Because of the spirochete's extreme thinness, it is difficult to detect by light microscopy; therefore, spirochetes are diagnosed by use of a specially adapted technique known as darkfield microscopy. Clinically, syphilis is divided into primary, secondary, and tertiary (or late) syphilis. In primary syphilis a hard chancre develops. This is a painless ulcer with an indurated base that is usually found on the vulva, vagina, or cervix. Secondary syphilis is the result of hematogenous dissemination of the spirochetes and thus is a systemic disease. There are a number of systemic symptoms depending on the major organs involved. The classic rash of secondary syphilis is red macules and papules over the palms of the hands and the soles of the feet. The manifestations of late syphilis include optic atrophy, tabes dorsalis, generalized paresis, aortic aneurysm, and gummas of the skin and bones.

348. The answer is d. *(Ransom 1997, pp 51–52.)* Primary genital herpes is characterized by pain, headaches, myalgias, and fever. Tender inguinal adenopathy is present and burning on urination can result in urinary retention. The diagnosis is generally made clinically, but viral cultures taken from one of the ulcers are the most accurate way of confirming the diagnosis. Onset of symptoms begins within 6 days of exposure, with initial symptoms lasting 2 to 6 wk. Oral acyclovir is the treatment of choice; it reduces viral shedding, significantly shortening healing time and reducing the number of days that the patient will remain symptomatic. Acyclovir ointment is no longer recommended. Herpes simplex virus type 1 (HSV-1) is seen in 13% to 40% of all pelvic herpetic infections. HSV-2 is more common. The herpes virus resides in the dorsal root ganglia of S2, S3, and S4. Recurrence is common, but the rate of recurrence can be significantly decreased with prolonged treatment with oral acyclovir.

349. The answer is d. *(Ransom 1997, pp 53–54.)* Condyloma acuminatum is a sexually transmitted disease caused by the human papillomavirus (HPV). For many years application of podophyllum was the treatment of choice for vulvar warts. Because podophyllum can produce peripheral neuropathy, bone marrow depression, and occasionally death, most physicians recommend the application of trichloroacetic acid to the vulva; however, because of systemic absorption, neither medication should be applied to extensive vaginal lesions. Laser surgery and cryotherapy result in high recurrence rates because of the difficulty of reaching all areas of the vagina. Since the vaginal condylomas are generally flat, optimal medical management includes the topical application of 5% 5-fluorouracil cream.

350. The answer is a. (_Ransom 1997, p 52._) The VDRL is a serologic test widely used to screen for syphilis. False positives appear in approximately 3% to 4% of all VDRL tests performed. If a positive test result is obtained, a physician first should ensure that the result is not due to a technical error and then should consider the various entities that result in false positives at the following rates: leprosy (8% to 28%), smallpox vaccination (1% to 2%), narcotic addiction (20% to 25%), and old age (10% of patients between 70 and 80 years of age). Atypical pneumonias have also resulted in false positives. The fluorescent treponemal antibody absorption (FTA-ABS) test, which is very specific, should be used with a borderline or suspected false positive VDRL test to confirm or refute this diagnosis.

351. The answer is b. (_Ransom 1997, p 53._) Lymphogranuloma venereum (LGV) is a chronic infection produced by _Chlamydia trachomatis_. The primary infection begins as a painless ulcer on the labia or vaginal vestibule; the patient usually consults the physician several weeks after the development of painful adenopathy in the inguinal and perirectal areas. Diagnosis can be established by culture or by demonstrating the presence of antibodies to _C. trachomatis_. The Frei skin test is no longer used because of its low sensitivity. The differential diagnosis includes syphilis, chancroid, granuloma inguinale, carcinoma, and herpes. Chancroid is a sexually transmitted disease caused by _Haemophilus ducreyi_ that produces a painful, tender ulceration of the vulva. Donovan bodies are present in patients with granuloma inguinale, which is caused by _Calymmatobacterium granulomatis_. Therapy for both granuloma inguinale and LGV is administration of tetracycline. Chancroid is successfully treated with either azithromycin or ceftriaxone.

352. The answer is c. (_Rock, 8/e, pp 1211–1213._) The most common cause of fecal incontinence is obstetric trauma with inadequate repair. The rectal sphincter can be completely lacerated, but as long as the patient retains a functional puborectalis sling, a high degree of continence will be maintained. Generally the patient is continent of formed stool but not of flatus. Other causes of fecal incontinence include senility, central nervous system (CNS) disease, rectal prolapse, diabetes, chronic diarrhea, and inflammatory bowel disease. While rectal prolapse, CNS disease, and senility are thus potential causes of this condition, they can be excluded by the history of the patient in the question. Approximately 20% of all diabetics complain of fecal incontinence. Therapy for fecal incontinence includes bulk-forming and antispasmodic agents, especially in those patients presenting with diarrhea. All caffeinated beverages should be stopped. Biofeedback and electrical stimulation of the rectal sphincter are other possible conservative treatments. Surgical repair of a defect is indicated when conservative measures fail, when the defect is large, or when symptoms warrant a more aggressive treatment approach.

353. The answer is a. (*Rock, 8/e, pp 375–378.*) Partial colpocleisis by the Le Fort procedure is reasonable for elderly patients who are not good candidates for vaginal hysterectomy and A&P (anterior and posterior) repair as treatment for vaginal and uterine prolapse. The technique involves partial denudation of opposing surfaces of the vaginal mucosa followed by surgical apposition, thereby resulting in partial obliteration of the vagina. Patients who are candidates for this procedure must have no evidence of cervical dysplasia or endometrial hyperplasia, have an atrophic endometrium, and no longer desire sexual function since the vaginal is essentially obliterated and there is no longer access to the cervix or uterus via the vagina. Urinary incontinence can be a side effect of this procedure, so care must be exercised in the denudation of vaginal mucosa near the bladder. In a patient who already has urinary incontinence, the Le Fort operation would be relatively contraindicated. An A&P repair essentially involves excision of redundant mucosa along the anterior and posterior walls of the vagina, at the same time strengthening the vaginal walls by suturing the laternal paravaginal fascia together in the midline.

354. The answer is a. (*Rock, 8/e, pp 951–962.*) All the factors mentioned in the question are commonly seen in patients with genital relaxation (with formation of an enterocele, rectocele, cystocele, or urethrocele, alone or in combination) and uterine prolapse. Undoubtedly, the most important factor is the actual quality of the tissue itself. In black and Asian patients there is a much lower incidence of uterine prolapse and enterocele formation in comparison with whites. Any factors that increase abdominal pressure can aggravate or further deteriorate the prolapse. Although the actual number of deliveries is probably not important, traumatic deliveries, especially those in which the rectal sphincter is lacerated or improperly repaired, have been associated with pelvic relaxation.

355. The answer is c. (*Mishell, 3/e, p 236. Rock, 8/e, pp 408–412.*) The most devastating injury to occur during laparoscopy is perforation of the aorta. Patients at high risk for vascular injury include thin, nulliparous women with well-developed abdominal musculature; the aorta may lie less than an inch below the skin in such women. Inadequate equipment and preparation, such as a dull trocar, inadequate pneumoperitoneum, or insertion of the trocar through a scar, all increase the likelihood of loss of control of the trocar and subsequent injury. A perpendicular entry also leaves less margin for error and a greater chance of hitting a vascular structure or bowel.

356. The answer is b. (*Scott, 8/e, pp 762–765.*) Most cases of urethral diverticula result from an infectious and not congenital etiology. This is demonstrated by the fact that most detailed urologic examinations of children are normal. Infections secondary to intercourse or other urinary tract infections may make the urethra more susceptible to trauma or stricture and result in dysuria, frequency, urgency, and incontinence.

357. The answer is d. (*Scott, 8/e, pp 770–777.*) There are many procedures that will provide successful correction of stress urinary incontinence. One of the abdominal procedures that successfully cures stress incontinence is the Marshall-Marchetti-Krantz (MMK) procedure, which involves the attachment of the periurethral tissue to the symphysis pubis. However, in approximately 3% of those patients undergoing the procedure, the painfully debilitating condition of osteitis pubis will develop. Treatment of this aseptic inflammation of the symphysis is suboptimal, and the course is usually chronic. An alternative—the Burch procedure—was therefore introduced; this involves the attachment of the periurethral tissue to Cooper's ligament. The incidences of urinary retention, recurrent urinary tract infections, and failure are essentially the same in the MMK and Burch procedures. Other procedures commonly employed in the treatment of stress incontinence are anterior repair and needle urethropexy (Stamey-Pererya procedure). The traditional anterior repair, or Kelly plication, has a 5-year failure rate of approximately 50%. The initial cure rate (90%) for the

Stamey-Pererya procedure appears to equal that of the Burch or MMK procedures.

358. The answer is e. (*Rock, 8/e, pp 1156–1157.*) This case presents a classic scenario for ureteral injury during hysterectomy. Recall that the ureters pass just under the uterine vessels as these course laterally from the uterus through the base of the broad ligament (see questions 291–295). As sutures are indiscriminately placed in this area when hemorrhage occurs, the risk of ureteral injury is high. Both ligation and crush injury of the ureter can occur, or the ureter can be included in a vascular pedicle and transected. Intraoperative recognition of these injuries requires a high index of suspicion. Many surgeons routinely identify the ureters during hysterectomy by opening the parietal peritoneum at the level of the round ligaments, and then dissecting down to the ureters, which adhere to the medially reflected peritoneum. Ligation or transection can be identified using intravenous indigo carmine or methylene blue, or cannulation via the ureteral ostia during cystoscopy or cystotomy. When ureteral ligation or transection is identified, the ligature is removed and either an indwelling stent with extraperitoneal drainage is placed, the ligated segment is resected and the ureter is reimplanted into the bladder, or the ligated segment is resected and an anastomosis is performed.

359. The answer is e. (*Rock, 8/e, pp 1156–1157.*) Implanting a severed ureter into the bladder is the procedure of choice, especially when the ureteral transection is near the bladder, as would be expected in this case. Following an injury to the ureter during surgery, a drain should be placed extraperitoneally, not intraperitoneally. If a polyethylene catheter is inserted, it should be placed above the site of injury so that urine is drained before arrival at the site of injury. Ureteroureteral anastomosis should be done only if reimplantation into the bladder is not feasible.

360. The answer is d. (*Mishell, 3/e, pp 577–578.*) As a catheter is introduced for performing a cystometrogram, measurement of residual urine is obtained. During the cystometrogram a normal first sensation is of fullness felt at 100 mL. Urge is felt at approximately 350, with maximum capacity at 450 mL. The primary reason to perform a cystometrogram is to rule out uninhibited detrusor contractions. The cystometrogram is a urodynamic test, and it cannot determine whether ureterovesical reflux exists. The degree of reflux can be evaluated with the voiding cystogram, a radiologic test.

361. The answer is e. *(Ransom 1997, p 53.)* The lesions shown in the figure accompanying the question are condyloma acuminatum, also known as venereal warts. This is a squamous lesion caused by a human papillomavirus (HPV). The lesion reveals a treelike growth microscopically with a mantle that shows marked acanthosis and parakeratosis. Treatment options include local excision, cryosurgery, application of podophyllum or trichloroacetic acid, and laser therapy, although podophyllin is not recommended for extensive disease because of toxicity (peripheral neuropathy). For intractable condyloma of the vagina, 5-fluorouracil can be employed. Vulvectomy is rarely indicated. A strong relationship between condyloma and intraepithelial neoplasia and carcinoma of the cervix has recently been demonstrated.

362. The answer is a. *(Mishell, 3/e, pp 629–631.)* Fungal cultures can confirm and identify the type of fungal organism. A wet smear for microscopic examination can miss a large percentage of fungal infections. Saline suspension is used to look for *Trichomonas vaginalis* organisms and for clue cells that are associated with *Gardnerella vaginalis* vaginitis. A bimanual pelvic examination is not helpful, and most discharges are of a white or yellowish color, so these would not help to identify the infecting organism.

363. The answer is c. *(Mishell, 3/e, pp 637–643.)* Persons at high risk for infection by human immunodeficiency virus (HIV) include homosexuals, bisexual males, women having sex with a bisexual or homosexual partner, intravenous drug users, and hemophiliacs. The virus can be transmitted through sexual contact, use of contaminated needles or blood products, and perinatal transmission from mother to child. The antibody titer usually becomes positive 6 to 12 wk after exposure, and the presence of the antibody provides no protection against acquired immunodeficiency syndrome (AIDS). Because of occasional delayed appearance of the antibody after initial exposure, it is important to follow up patients for 1 year after exposure.

364–368. The answers are 364-d, 365-a, 366-b, 367-b, 368-e. *(Scott, 8/e, pp 583–586.)* Many cases of nonspecific vaginitis are caused by *Gard-*

nerella vaginalis. Women with this infection usually complain of a characteristically malodorous, grayish vaginal discharge. On wet mounts, the diagnosis is made by visualizing clue cells, which are epithelial cells with large numbers of adherent coccobacilli. The recommended treatment is ampicillin, although vaginal sulfa creams are also effective.

Besides diabetes mellitus, other predisposing factors of candidiasis include pregnancy, the use of antibiotics, immunosuppressive medications, and possibly oral contraceptives. Affected women usually complain of severe pruritus and a thick, cheeselike vaginal discharge. Wet mounts show characteristic yeast cells and hyphae. The primary mode of treatment is the vaginal application of an antifungal agent, or single-dose regimens of oral antifungal agents.

Trichomonas vaginalis classically gives rise to a yellowish, frothy discharge that is foul-smelling and causes pruritus. The pathognomonic "strawberry spots," which consist of punctate hemorrhagic spots on the vaginal or cervical mucosa, can sometimes be seen. The diagnosis is made by observing the characteristic motile protozoan on wet mounts. The mainstay of treatment is oral metronidazole, either in a single dose of 2 g or 250 mg three times a day for 7 to 10 days. Metronidazole has a disulfiram-like effect, and women taking it should refrain from consumption of alcohol. Vaginal suppositories of clotrimazole, 100 mg once a day for 7 days, are also effective and are preferred by some because of carcinogenicity in rodents treated with metronidazole.

Postmenopausal women who present with symptoms like itching, irritation secondary to dryness, and dyspareunia often have atrophic (senile) vaginitis. Owing to the lack of estrogen, the vaginal mucosa becomes very thin, friable, and easily irritable. This condition responds well to either oral intake of estrogen or local application of estrogen creams.

While the Bartholin's glands, endocervical glands, and fallopian tubes can all be infected by *Neisseria gonorrhoeae,* infection of the vaginal mucosa by this organism is uncommon. Hence vaginal discharge and vaginitis are not caused by *Neisseria.* However, gonococcal cervicitis can occur, and the resulting blood-tinged mucopurulent discharge, if profuse, may initially appear as an atypical vaginitis discharge.

369–372. The answers are 369-d, 370-a, 371-c, 372-e. *(Mishell, 3/e, pp 613–623. Ransom 1997, p 52.)* The treatment for primary syphilis is benzathine penicillin, 2.4 million U intramuscularly. For those patients who are allergic to penicillin, tetracycline may be given. In a patient with acute salpingitis with culture-proven chlamydia who does not respond to conventional therapy, tetracycline should be added. Drugs active against *Bacteroides fragilis* include cefoxitin, clindamycin, metronidazole, and chloramphenicol. Many feel that patients presenting with pelvic inflammatory disease should be given a drug that has anaerobic coverage and that the regimen of penicillin and gentamicin is not adequate. Uncomplicated gonorrheal infections are generally treated with oral tetracycline, amoxicillin/ ampicillin, or aqueous procaine penicillin. In patients with penicillinase-producing *Neisseria gonorrhoeae,* spectinomycin 2 g intramuscularly is given in a single injection. An alternative medication is cefoxitin. Spectinomycin and cefoxitin are ineffective in pharyngeal infections.

ENDOCRINOLOGY AND INFERTILITY

Questions

DIRECTIONS: Each item below contains a question or incomplete statement followed by suggested responses. Select the **one best** response to each question.

373. A 39-year-old woman, gravida 3, para 3, complains of severe, progressive secondary dysmenorrhea and menorrhagia. Pelvic examination demonstrates a tender, diffusely enlarged uterus with no adnexal tenderness. Results of endometrial biopsy are normal. This patient most likely has

a. Endometriosis
b. Endometritis
c. Adenomyosis
d. Uterine sarcoma
e. Leiomyoma

374. The most important indication for surgical repair of a double uterus, such as a septate or bicornuate uterus, is

a. Habitual abortion
b. Dysmenorrhea
c. Menometrorrhagia
d. Dyspareunia
e. Premature delivery

375. In an amenorrheic patient who has had pituitary ablation for a craniopharyngioma, which of the following regimens is most likely to result in an ovulatory cycle?

a. Clomiphene citrate
b. Pulsatile infusion of gonadotropin-releasing hormone (GnRH)
c. Continuous infusion of GnRH
d. Human menopausal or recombinant gonadotropin
e. Human menopausal or recombinant gonadotropin followed by human chorionic gonadotropin (hCG)

376. Studies of family histories involving mothers and daughters with endometriosis suggest which type of inheritance pattern?

a. No genetic basis
b. Autosomal dominant
c. Sex-linked
d. Polygenic or multifactorial
e. Autosomal recessive

377. Follicle-stimulating hormone is elaborated by

a. Chromophobe cells of the adenohypophysis
b. Basophilic cells of the adenohypophysis
c. Acidophilic cells of the adenohypophysis
d. Theca interna cells
e. The posterior pituitary

378. In the evaluation of a 26-year-old patient with 4 mo of secondary amenorrhea, you order serum prolactin and β-hCG assays. The pregnancy test is positive and the prolactin comes back at 100 ng/mL (normal <25 ng/ml in this assay). This patient requires

a. Routine obstetric care
b. Computed tomography (CT) scan of her sella turcica to rule out pituitary adenoma
c. Repeat measurements of serum prolactin to ensure that values do not increase over 300 ng/mL
d. Bromocriptine to suppress prolactin
e. Evaluation for possible hypothyroidism

379. Which of the following medications is used as first-line therapy in the treatment of endometriosis?

a. Unopposed estrogens
b. Dexamethasone
c. Danazol
d. Gonadotropins
e. Parlodel

380. A 28-year-old nulligravid patient complains of bleeding between her periods and increasingly heavy menses. Over the past 9 mo she has had two dilation and curettages (D&Cs), which have failed to resolve her symptoms, and oral contraceptives and antiprostaglandins have not decreased the abnormal bleeding. Of the following options, which is most appropriate at his time?

a. Perform a hysterectomy
b. Perform hysteroscopy
c. Perform endometrial ablation
d. Treat with a GnRH agonist
e. Start the patient on a high-dose progestational agent

381. Danazol used in the treatment of endometriosis causes which of the following changes within the endometrium and endometriosis tissue?

a. Aplasia
b. Atrophy
c. Hyperplasia
d. Neoplasia
e. Inflammation

382. Which of the following conditions can be diagnosed with a hysterosalpingogram?

a. Endometriosis
b. Hydrosalpinx
c. Subserous fibroids
d. Minimal pelvic adhesions
e. Ovarian cyst

383. The presentation of Asherman syndrome typically involves

a. Hypomenorrhea
b. Oligomenorrhea
c. Menorrhagia
d. Metrorrhagia
e. Dysmenorrhea

384. During the evaluation of secondary amenorrhea in a 24-year-old woman, hyperprolactinemia is diagnosed. Which of the following conditions could cause increased circulating prolactin concentration and amenorrhea in this patient?

a. Stress
b. Primary hyperthyroidism
c. Anorexia nervosa
d. Congenital adrenal hyperplasia
e. Polycystic ovarian disease

385. Premenopausal peripheral conversion of estrogen precursors in the obese patient results in the formation of

a. Estriol
b. Estradiol
c. Estrone
d. Androstenedione
e. Dehydroepiandrosterone

386. Androgens are predominantly produced in the adrenal gland or ovary. The most clinically useful hormonal measurement to differentiate between ovarian and adrenal production is

a. Ratio of testosterone to free testosterone
b. Dehydroepiandrosterone sulfate (DHAS)
c. Dehydroepiandrosterone
d. Dehydrotestosterone (DHT)
e. Androstenedione

387. You are evaluating a 13-year-old girl with delayed puberty and short stature. Human growth hormone (hGH) assay done on a fasting blood sample suggests hGH deficiency. You plan to schedule a provocative test of hGH release. Which of the following will stimulate hGH release?

a. Lysine
b. L-dopa
c. Glucose
d. Bed rest
e. Gonadotropin-releasing hormone

388. Varicoceles appear to cause male infertility by

a. Interfering with sperm production
b. Blocking epididymal sperm motility activation
c. Increasing the likelihood of sperm antibody formation
d. Interfering with sperm movement through cervical mucus
e. None of the above

389. The presence of a uterus and fallopian tubes in an otherwise phenotypically normal male is due to

a. Lack of müllerian inhibiting factor
b. Lack of testosterone
c. Increased levels of estrogens
d. 46,XX karyotype
e. Presence of ovarian tissue early in embryonic development

390. Which of the following factors is produced primarily in the corpus luteum?

a. Activin
b. Follistatin
c. Epidermal growth factor
d. Inhibin
e. Relaxin

391. In the workup of the infertile couple, a sperm penetration assay is done for which of the following purposes?

a. To assess tubal patency
b. To replace a regular sperm analysis
c. To evaluate ejaculatory disorders
d. To determine the fertilizing capacity of sperm
e. To assess penetration of sperm through cervical mucus

392. Luteal phase defects are ovulatory disorders that can be a cause of infertility. Which of the following studies performed in the second half of the menstrual cycle is helpful in making this diagnosis?

a. Serum estradiol levels
b. Urinary pregnanetriol levels
c. Endometrial biopsy
d. Serum follicle-stimulating hormone (FSH) levels
e. Serum luteinizing hormone (LH) levels

393. Progesterone production by the placenta during a normal pregnancy is dependent upon which of the following?

a. Uteroplacental perfusion
b. Chorionic gonadotropin levels
c. Maternal low-density lipoprotein (LDL) cholesterol
d. The fetal adrenal gland
e. A live fetus

394. A 45-year-old woman who has had two normal pregnancies 15 and 18 years ago presents with the complaint of amenorrhea for 7 mo. She expresses the desire to become pregnant again. After exclusion of pregnancy, which of the following tests is next indicated in the evaluation of this patient's amenorrhea?

a. Hysterosalpingogram
b. Endometrial biopsy
c. Thyroid function tests
d. Testosterone and DHAS levels
e. LH and FSH levels

395. Which of the following ovarian actions is attributable to LH during the follicular phase of the ovarian cycle?

a. Stimulation of the production of primordial follicles
b. Stimulation of the production of GnRH by the hypothalamus
c. Stimulation of the production of estrogen by thecal cells
d. Stimulation of the production of androgen by thecal cells
e. Stimulation of granulose cell mitosis and division

396. A 22-year-old woman consults you for treatment of hirsutism. She is obese and has facial acne and hirsutism on her face and periareolar regions and a male escutcheon. Serum LH level is 35 mIU/ml and FSH is 9 mIU/ml. Androstenedione and testosterone levels are mildly elevated, but serum DHAS is normal. The patient does not wish to conceive at this time. Which of the following single agents is the most appropriate treatment of her condition?

a. Oral contraceptives
b. Corticosteroids
c. GnRH
d. Parlodel
e. Wedge resection

397. Which of the following is not a physiologic action of parathyroid hormone?

a. Conversion of 25-hydroxyvitamin-D to 1,25-dihydroxyvitamin-D
b. Bone resorption
c. Renal tubular resorption
d. Increased intestinal absorption
e. Inhibition of production of 1α-hydroxylase

398. An 18-year-old college student who has recently become sexually active is seen for severe primary dysmenorrhea. She does not want to get pregnant, and has failed to obtain resolution with heating pads and mild analgesics. Which of the following medications is most appropriate for this patient?

a. Prostaglandin inhibitors
b. Narcotic analgesics
c. Oxytocin
d. Oral contraceptives
e. Luteal progesterone

399. Retrograde menstruation is the most accepted mechanism to explain the etiology of endometriosis. Another theory suggests that some stimulus causes metaplasia of the celomic epithelium, leading to endometriosis. Endometriosis in which of the following patients is evidence of the celomic metaplasia theory of causation?

a. A patient with endometriosis in an episiotomy scar
b. A patient with endometriosis of the subarachnoid space
c. A patient with endometriosis in the lung
d. A patient with müllerian agenesis
e. A patient with endometriosis in a laparoscopy scar

400. A 19-year-old patient presents to your office with primary amenorrhea. She has normal breast and public hair development, but the uterus and vagina are absent. Diagnostic possibilities include

a. XYY syndrome
b. Gonadal dysgenesis
c. Müllerian agenesis
d. Klinefelter syndrome
e. Turner syndrome

401. Which of the following medications is most useful for the treatment of premenstrual syndrome?

a. Progesterone
b. Anxiolytics
c. Vitamins
d. Antiprostaglandins
e. Selective serotonin reuptake inhibitors (SSRIs)

402. A 31-year-old patient complains of increasingly prolonged and heavy periods. Hysteroscopy may aid in the diagnosis by identifying

a. Submucous myoma
b. Subserous myoma
c. Endometrial septum
d. Luteal phase defect
e. Tubal occlusion

403. A 19-year-old woman is a gymnast and runner. She exercises approximately 6 h per day. Amenorrhea in this patient is most likely associated with

a. Decreased β-lipotropin
b. Increased β-endorphins
c. Decreased prolactin
d. Increased gonadotropins
e. Decreased growth hormone

404. A 23-year-old woman presents for evaluation of a 7-mo history of amenorrhea. Examination discloses bilateral galactorrhea and normal breast and pelvic examinations. Pregnancy test is negative. Which of the following classes of medication is a possible cause of her condition?

a. Antiestrogens
b. Gonadotropins
c. Phenothiazines
d. Prostaglandins
e. GnRH analogs

405. Which of the following pubertal events in girls is not estrogen dependent?

a. Menses
b. Vaginal cornification
c. Hair growth
d. Reaching adult height
e. Production of cervical mucus

406. A 9-year-old girl has breast and pubic hair development. Evaluation demonstrates a pubertal response to a gonadotropin-releasing hormone (GnRH) stimulation test, and a prominent increase in luteinizing hormone (LH) pulses during sleep. These findings are characteristic of patients with

a. Theca cell tumors
b. Iatrogenic sexual precocity
c. Premature thelarche
d. Granulosa cell tumors
e. Constitutional precocious puberty

Items 407–412

Match the gonadotropin actions during specific phases of the menstrual cycle (a–e) with the numbered actions or ovarian follicle characteristics below.

a. LH in the follicular phase
b. LH in the periovulatory phase
c. LH in the luteal phase
d. FSH in the follicular phase
e. FSH in the luteal phase

407. Receptors are initially present only on theca cells

408. Causes granulosa cells to aromatize androstenedione and testosterone to estrone and estradiol, respectively

409. Induces the appearance of LH receptors on granulosa cells

410. Induces the appearance of FSH receptors on granulosa cells

411. Causes proliferation of granulosa cells

412. Stimulates steroid production from the corpus luteum

413. Which of the following findings characterize a normal semen sample?

a. Agglutination
b. 35 million/ml sperm concentration
c. 5% normal sperm morphology
d. 10% progressive sperm motility
e. A volume of 1 mL

DIRECTIONS: Each group of questions below consists of lettered options followed by numbered items. For each numbered item, select the appropriate lettered option(s). Each lettered option may be used once, more than once, or not at all. **Choose exactly the number of options indicated following each item.**

Items 414–418

Match each hysterosalpingogram with the correct description. (SELECT 1 DESCRIPTION)

a. Bilateral hydrosalpinx
b. Unilateral hydrosalpinx with intrauterine adhesions
c. Unilateral hydrosalpinx with a normal uterine cavity
d. Bilateral proximal occlusion
e. Salpingitis isthmica nodosa
f. Bilateral normal spillage

414.

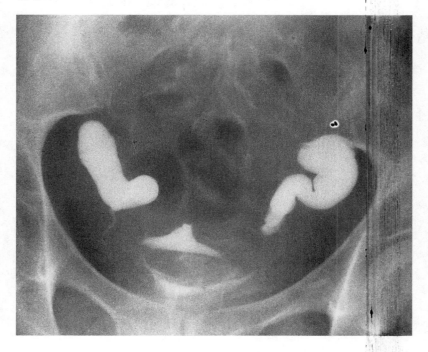

415.

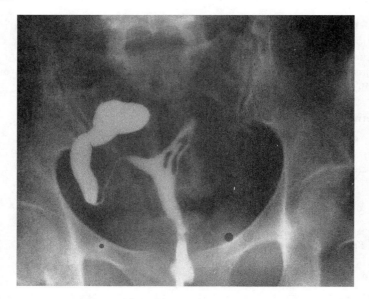

416.

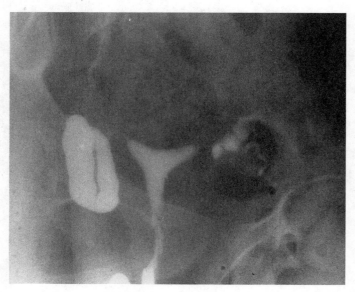

417.

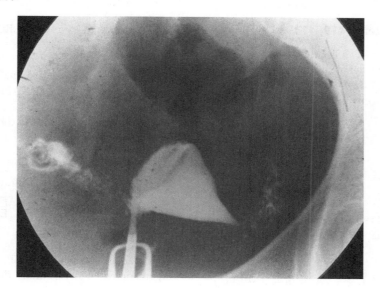

418.

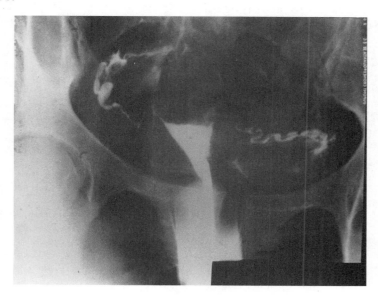

Items 419–423

For each evaluation, select the most appropriate day of a normal 28-day menstrual cycle for a woman with 5 day menstrual cycles.

a. Day 3
b. Day 8
c. Day 14
d. Day 21
e. Day 26

419. Endometrial biopsy for evaluation of infertility (**SELECT 1 DAY**)

420. Postcoital test (**SELECT 1 DAY**)

421. Hysterosalpingogram (**SELECT 1 DAY**)

422. Determination of serum progesterone level to document ovulation (**SELECT 1 DAY**)

423. Gonadotropin evaluation (**SELECT 1 DAY**)

Items 424–428

Match each action listed below with the appropriate enzyme.

a. Adenylcyclase
b. 5α-reductase
c. 17β-hydroxysteroid dehydrogenase
d. cholesterol desmolase
e. 21-dehydroxylase

424. Is activated by LH (**SELECT 1 ENZYME**)

425. Converts androstenedione to testosterone (**SELECT 1 ENZYME**)

426. Converts testosterone to dihydrotestosterone (**SELECT 1 ENZYME**)

427. Catalyzes the first step in the production of hormonal steroids from cholesterol (**SELECT 1 ENZYME**)

428. Causes massive adrenal enlargement when congenitally deficient, is associated with poor survival of affected infants, and can lead to the formation of female genitalia in genotypically male infants (**SELECT 1 ENZYME**)

ENDOCRINOLOGY
AND INFERTILITY

Answers

373. The answer is c. *(Mishell, 3/e, pp 537–540.)* Adenomyosis is a condition in which normal endometrial glands grow into the myometrium. Symptomatic disease primarily occurs in multiparous women over the age of 35 years, compared to endometriosis in which onset is considerably younger. Patients with adenomyosis complain of dysmenorrhea and menorrhagia, and the classical examination findings include a tender, symmetrically enlarged uterus without adnexal tenderness. Although patients with endometriosis can have similar complaints, the physical examination of these patients more commonly reveals a fixed, retroverted uterus, adnexal tenderness and scarring, and tenderness along the uterosacral ligaments. Leiomyoma is the most common pelvic tumor, but the majority are asymptomatic and the uterus is irregular in shape. Patients with endometritis can present with abnormal bleeding, but endometrial biopsies show an inflammatory pattern. Uterine sarcoma is rare, and presents in older women with postmenopausal bleeding and nontender uterine enlargement.

374. The answer is a. *(Speroff, 6/e, pp 145–149.)* Habitual abortion is the most important indication for surgical treatment of women who have a double uterus. The abortion rate in women who have a double uterus is two to three times greater than that of the general population. Therefore, women who present with habitual abortion should be evaluated to detect a possible double uterus. Hysterosalpingography, hysteroscopy, ultrasound, CT, and magnetic resonance imaging (MRI) are all potentially useful imaging modalities in this investigation. Dysmenorrhea, premature delivery, dyspareunia, and menometrorrhagia are other, less important indicators for surgical intervention.

375. The answer is e. *(Mishell, 3/e, pp 1059–1063.)* This patient would be unable to produce endogenous gonadotropin, since her pituitary has been ablated. The patient will therefore need to be given exogenous gonadotropin in the form of human menopausal gonadotropin (hMG), which contains an extract of urine from postmenopausal women with follicle-stimulating hormone (FSH) and luteinizing hormone (LH) in various ratios. Recombinant human FSH (rhFSH) is now also available. Carefully timed administration of hCG, which takes the place of an endogenous LH surge, will be needed to complete oocyte maturation and induce ovulation. Clomiphene citrate acts by competing with endogenous circulating estrogens for estrogen-binding sites in the hypothalamus. Therefore, it blocks the normal negative feedback of the endogenous estrogens and stimulates release of endogenous GnRH. However, the pituitary will not respond in this patient. Endogenous or exogenous GnRH cannot stimulate the release of FSH or LH in this woman because the pituitary gland is nonfunctional.

376. The answer is d. (*Mishell, 3/e, pp 517–520.*) Studies have shown a predisposition to endometriosis in daughters whose mothers had the disease, and women whose sisters have endometriosis are more likely to have it as well. Women who have a family history of endometriosis are likely to develop the disease earlier in life and have more advanced disease than women whose first-degree relatives are free of the disease. The predisposition to develop endometriosis is transmitted via a polygenic or multifactorial inheritance pattern.

377. The answer is b. (*Mishell, 3/e, p 1050.*) Luteinizing hormone (LH) and follicle-stimulating hormone (FSH) are synthesized in, stored in, and secreted from the basophilic cells of the adenohypophysis (anterior pituitary). It appears that a single cell type makes both LH and FSH. In addition, GnRH, elaborated by the hypothalamus, is responsible for secretion of both pituitary gonadotropins.

378. The answer is a. (*Mishell, 3/e, pp 1070–1071.*) There is a marked increase in levels of serum prolactin during gestation to over 10 times those values found in nonpregnant women. If this woman were not pregnant, the prolactin value could easily explain the amenorrhea and further evaluation of hyperprolactinemia would be necessary. The physiologic significance of increasing prolactin in pregnancy appears to involve preparation of the breasts for lactation.

379. The answer is c. (*Speroff, 6/e, pp 1064–1065.*) Medical treatment of endometriosis currently involves a selection of four medications—oral contraceptive pills (OCPs), continuous progestins, danazol, and GnRH analogs. Surgery, both via a laparoscopic approach and laparotomy, is also used to treat endometriosis. One of the first medical treatments for endometriosis was the uninterrupted (acyclic) administration of high-dose birth-control pills for prolonged periods of time. Today this regimen is not used as often as it once was. Progestin therapy can lead to subjective and objective improvement in patients with endometriosis. Problems with continuous progestin therapy include breakthrough bleeding and depression. Overall, however, the side effects of progestin therapy are less than those seen with other treatments in most patients. Progestin therapy is generally reserved for patients who do not desire fertility. Danazol is an isoxazol derivative of 17α-ethinyl testosterone; it has been characterized as a pseudomenopausal treatment for endometriosis. Side effects include weight gain, edema, decreased breast size, acne, and other menopausal symptoms. GnRH agonists are the most recent addition to our armamentarium against endometriosis. These agents produce a medical oophorectomy. Collaborative studies have confirmed that fertility rates and symptom relief are similar between GnRH analogs and other medications. At the present time, conservative surgery compares favorably with administration of danazol in the management of mild to moderate endometriosis. Surgery is definitely indicated in patients with severe disease, those who fail hormonal therapy, or in the older infertile patient. Dexamethasone is not a treatment for endometriosis, and unopposed estrogen therapy would probably exacerbate the disease. Gonadotropins are used for ovulation induction, and parlodel is a dopamine agonist used in the treatment of hyperprolactinemia.

380. The answer is b. (*Mishell, 3/e, pp 229–232.*) In patients with abnormal bleeding who are not responding to standard therapy, hysteroscopy should be performed. Hysteroscopy can rule out endometrial polyps or small fibroids, which, if present, can be resected. In patients with heavy abnormal bleeding who no longer desire fertility, an endometrial ablation can be performed. If a patient had completed child bearing and was having significant abnormal bleeding, a hysteroscopy rather than a hysterectomy would still be the procedure of choice to rule out easily treatable disease. Treatment with a GnRH agonist would only temporarily relieve symptoms.

381. The answer is b. (*Speroff, 6/e, pp 1064–1065.*) Danazol is a progestational compound derived from testosterone that is used to treat endometriosis. It induces a pseudomenopause but does not alter basal gonadotropin levels. It appears to act as an antiestrogen and causes endometrial atrophy. Cyclic menses return almost immediately upon withdrawal of danazol. It is felt that the endometrium is poorly developed with danazol use and that three menstrual cycles should be allowed to pass before conception so as to avoid a higher risk of spontaneous abortion, which could result from implantation in this poorly developed endometrium.

382. The answer is b. (*Speroff, 6/e, pp 1025–1027.*) A hysterosalpingogram is a procedure in which 3 to 6 mL of either an oil- or water-soluble contrast medium is injected through the cervix in a retrograde fashion to outline the uterine cavity and fallopian tubes. Spill of contrast medium into the peritoneal cavity proves patency of the fallopian tubes. By outlining the uterine cavity, abnormalities such as bicornuate or septate uterus, uterine polyps, or submucous myomas can be diagnosed, while tubal opacification allows identification of such conditions as salpingitis isthmica nodosum and hydrosalpinx. However, pelvic abnormalities outside the uterine cavity and fallopian tube (such as subserous fibroids, ovarian tumors, endometriosis or minimal pelvic adhesions) are possibly not visible with this study, and hence a false-negative report could be generated. Some studies have shown a therapeutic effect resulting in an increased rate of pregnancy in the months immediately following the hysterosalpingogram.

383. The answer is a. (*Speroff, 6/e, p 440.*) Ovulation is not affected in Asherman syndrome. Because of the decreased amount of functional endometrium, progressive hypomenorrhea (lighter menstrual flow) or amenorrhea is common. The best diagnostic study is the hysterosalpingogram under fluoroscopy. Hysteroscopy with lysis of adhesions is the treatment of choice. Prophylactic antibiotics may improve success rates.

384. The answer is a. (*Speroff, 6/e, pp 461–464.*) In anorexia nervosa, prolactin, thyroid-stimulating hormone (TSH), and thyroxine levels are normal, FSH and LH levels are low, and cortisol levels are elevated. Prolactin is under the control of prolactin inhibiting factor (PIF), which is produced in the hypothalamus. Many drugs (e.g., the phenothiazines), stress, hypothalamic lesions, stalk lesions, and stalk compression decrease PIF. In hypothyroidism, elevated TRH acts as a prolactin-releasing hormone to cause release of prolactin from the pituitary; hyperthyroidism is not associated with hyperprolactinemia. There are many other conditions, such as acromegaly and pregnancy, that are associated with elevated prolactin levels. Hyperandrogenic conditions such as congenital adrenal hyperplasia or polycystic ovarian disease are not typically associated with hyperprolactinemia.

385. The answer is c. *(Speroff, 6/e, pp 656–660.)* In premenopausal adult women, most of the estrogen in the body is derived from ovarian secretion of estradiol, but a significant portion comes also from the extraglandular conversion of androstenedione to estrone. To a lesser extent testosterone conversion to estradiol also contributes to the estrogen milieu. Muscle and adipose tissue are the major sites of aromatization. When there is an increase in fat cells, as in obese persons, estrogen levels will be higher, because adipose tissue exhibits a greater aromatization of androstenedione to estrone than does muscle.

386. The answer is b. *(Speroff, 6/e, pp 526–527.)* Testosterone is produced both in the adrenal gland and the ovary, with each contributing approximately 25%. Fifty percent of testosterone production is from the peripheral conversion of androstenedione. Androstenedione is produced in equal amounts by the adrenal gland and the ovary. Although 90% of the dehydroepiandrosterone is produced in the adrenal gland, the ovary contributes approximately 10%. Dehydroepiandrosterone sulfate (DHAS) is produced entirely by the adrenal gland. While DHAS is elevated slightly in patients with polycystic ovarian disease, significant elevations occur with adrenal tumors or adrenal hyperplasia. Differentiation is assessed by the patient's ability to suppress DHAS after dexamethasone therapy.

387. The answer is b. *(Mishell, 3/e, p 95.)* A single fasting blood sample, while sufficient to screen for growth hormone (GH) deficiency, is not diagnostic of this condition. Many believe that inadequate GH secretion is not established until the absence of significant release is documented following the use of several provocative stimuli. Strenuous exercise has been recognized as a potent physiologic stimulus to GH secretion. The L-dopa, insulin tolerance, and arginine tolerance tests all assess GH secretion.

388. The answer is c. *(Keye, pp 559–561, 629–637.)* The incidence of varicoceles in the general population is about 15%, but 40% of males with infertility are found to have varicoceles. Because of the anatomy and physiology, varicoceles are more likely to occur on the left side. There is no correlation between the size of the varix and prognosis for fertility. The characteristic stress pattern seen with varicoceles is decreased number of sperm, decreased motility, and increased abnormal forms. How the varicocele causes abnormal semen quality, and the relationship between varicocele, semen abnormalities, and male infertility (especially when semen quality appears normal) is unclear.

389. The answer is a. (*Speroff, 6/e, pp 124–125, 441–442.*) Remember that the müllerian structures appear during embryonic development in both males and females. Female gonads do not secrete müllerian inhibiting factor (MIF) and the müllerian structures persist. Male testes secrete MIF, which causes regression of müllerian structures. Anything that prevents MIF secretion in genetic males will result in persistence of müllerian structures into the postnatal period. Persons who appear to be normal males but who possess a uterus and tubes have such a failure of müllerian inhibiting factor. Their karyotype is 46,XY, testes are present, and testosterone production is normal. When the testes are located intraabdominally, orchidectomy is required to prevent malignant degeneration in these ectopic gonads.

390. The answer is e. (*Speroff, 6/e, pp 119, 230–237.*) There are numerous nonsteroidal factors produced by the ovary that affect endocrine, autocrine, and paracrine regulation of normal ovarian function. Relaxin produced by the corpus luteum inhibits uterine contractions and aids in remodeling of the reproductive tract. Inhibin, activin, and follistatin are all produced from identical subunits throughout follicular and luteal phases of the ovarian cycle; inhibin and follistatin suppress FSH release, while activin stimulates FSH release. Epidermal growth factor is mitogenic to the granulosa cells but inhibits steroidogenesis. Oxytocin modulates progesterone secretion and regulates the life span of the corpus luteum.

391. The answer is d. (*Speroff, 6/e, p 1081.*) The sperm penetration assay determines the capacity of human sperm to penetrate hamster ova pretreated by removal of the zona pellucida (which blocks penetration by another species' sperm). The presence of a sperm head within the egg is considered a sign of penetration. As this is a functional test of the fertilizing ability of the sperm, the results do not always correlate with the sperm count or the postcoital test. This test may, therefore, complement semen analysis. Ejaculatory disorders are evaluated by semen analysis, urinalysis (for sperm), and a detailed history of sexual function. Tubal patency can be evaluated by a hysterosalpingogram (HSG) or laparoscopy. Sperm–cervical mucus interaction, and by inference the ability of sperm to penetrate through the cervical mucus, is assessed by the postcoital (Sims-Huhner) test; additional in vitro tests can be done to further evaluate sperm mucus interaction and barriers to sperm penetration if indicated.

392. The answer is c. *(Speroff, 6/e, pp 1031–1033.)* An abnormal luteal phase is defined as ovulation with a poor progestational effect in the second half of the cycle. Luteal function is usually evaluated at the endometrium, which is inadequately prepared for embryo implantation. Endometrial biopsy is crucial to the diagnosis of this defect because the endometrium will be out of phase with the time of cycle in these patients. For example, a biopsy taken on day 26 of the cycle will resemble endometrium of day 22 because of decreased progesterone stimulation. Progesterone levels in the midluteal phase less than 7 ng/mL are suggestive of a luteal phase defect but not diagnostic. Pregnanetriol is a breakdown product of 17-hydroxyprogesterone, and levels are not helpful in diagnosing this condition. Determination of the level of pregnanediol, which is a metabolic product of progesterone excreted in the urine, is helpful. Serum luteinizing hormone levels have no correlation with the presence of luteal phase defect.

393. The answer is c. *(Speroff, 6/e, pp 276–283.)* Major functions of progesterone produced during pregnancy include preparation of the endometrium for implantation, modification of the maternal immunologic response so that fetal antigens are tolerated, and serving as the precursor for fetal adrenal glucocorticoid and mineralocorticoid synthesis. Progesterone is produced exclusively by the corpus luteum until about 10 wk of pregnancy, with a period of shared production from about 7 to 10 wk. Indeed, during the first trimester, serum progesterone levels can be used to differentiate normal intrauterine pregnancies from abnormal or ectopic ones. The precursor for placental progesterone is maternal LDL cholesterol, the lipoprotein component of which provides amino acids for the fetus. This production appears to be independent of external trophic control, and does not depend upon fetal viability or uteroplacental perfusion. This is in contrast to estrogen production during pregnancy, which is directly under the control of the fetus. In fact, production of estriol (an estrogen found exclusively during pregnancy) involves pregnenolone as the direct precursor for a sequence of steps in the fetal adrenal, fetal liver, and placenta. Estrogens during pregnancy influence fetal adrenal function, progesterone production, uteroplacental blood flow, and breast development. The endocrinology of pregnancy is a complex topic that has considerable impact upon current obstetrical practice. For example, if something interferes with corpus luteum function during early pregnancy (for example, removal of a hemorrhagic corpus luteum cyst), supplemental progesterone is required until about 10 wk gestation, but not thereafter. Also, maternal serum estriol levels (part of the maternal serum triple screen) are used clinically to evaluate fetal well-being, since estriol production is dependent upon fetal adrenal and hepatic function.

394. The answer is e. *(Ransom 1997, p 136. Speroff, 6/e, pp 444–448, 651–656.)* This patient has secondary amenorrhea, which rules out abnormalities associated with primary amenorrhea such as chromosomal abnormalities and congenital müllerian abnormalities. The most common reason for amenorrhea in a woman of reproductive age is pregnancy, which should be evaluated first. Other possibilities include chronic endometritis or scarring of the endometrium (Asherman syndrome), hypothyroidism, and ovarian failure. The latter is the most likely diagnosis in a woman at this age. In addition, emotional stress, extreme weight loss, and adrenal cortisol insufficiency can bring about secondary amenorrhea. A hysterosalpingogram is part of an infertility workup that may demonstrate Asherman syndrome, but it is not indicated until premature ovarian failure has been excluded. Persistently elevated gonadotropin levels (especially when accompanied by low serum estradiol levels) are diagnostic of ovarian failure.

395. The answer is d. *(Speroff, 6/e, pp 206–209.)* The gonadotropins (FSH and LH) are glycoproteins that act on the gonads and not backward to the hypothalamus. In women, FSH stimulates the production of one or more primordial follicles and LH induces thecal cells in the ovary to produce androgen, which is converted to estrogen by aromatase in granulosa cells under the stimulus of FSH.

396. The answer is a. *(Speroff, 6/e, p 544.)* This patient has polycystic ovarian syndrome (PCOS), diagnosed by the clinical picture, abnormally high LH-to-FSH ratio (which should normally be approximately 1:1), and elevated androgens but normal DHAS. DHAS is a marker of adrenal androgen production; when normal it essentially excludes adrenal sources of hyperandrogenism. Several medications have been used to treat hirsutism associated with PCOS. For many years contraceptives were the most frequently used agents; they can suppress hair growth in up to two-thirds of treated patients. They act by directly suppressing ovarian steroid production and increasing hepatic binding globulin production, which binds circulating hormone and lowers the concentration of metabolically active (free, unbound) androgen. However, clinical improvement can take as long as 6 mo to manifest. Other medications that have shown promise include medroxyprogesterone acetate, spironolactone, cimetidine, and GnRH agonists, which suppress ovarian steroid production. However, GnRH analogs are expensive and have been associated with significant bone demineralization after only 6 mo of therapy in some patients. Surgical wedge resection is no longer considered an appropriate therapy for PCOS given the success of pharmacologic agents and the ovarian adhesions that were frequently associated with this surgery.

397. The answer is e. (*Mishell, 3/e, p 1170.*) Parathyroid hormone (PTH) maintains calcium homeostasis by raising serum calcium levels. It does so by increasing bone absorption (liberating calcium from skeletal stores), renal tubular reabsorption of calcium, and absorption of calcium from the gastrointestinal (GI) tract. In order to increase absorption from the GI tract, PTH increases production of the enzyme 1-α-hydroxylase. This enzyme aids in the conversion of 25-hydroxyvitamin D to 1,25-dihydroxyvitamin D.

398. The answer is d. (*Mishell, 3/e, pp 1011–1023.*) Conservative measures for treating dysmenorrhea include heating pads, mild analgesics, sedatives or antispasmodic drugs, and outdoor exercise. In patients with dysmenorrhea there is a significantly higher than normal concentration of prostaglandins in the endometrium and menstrual fluid. Prostaglandin synthase inhibitors such as indomethacin, naproxen, ibuprofen, and mefenamic acid are very effective in these patients. However, for patients with dysmenorrhea who are sexually active, oral contraceptives will provide needed protection from unwanted pregnancy and generally alleviate the dysmenorrhea. The OCPs minimize endometrial prostaglandin production during the concurrent administration of estrogen and progestin.

399. The answer is d. (*Speroff, 6/e, pp 1057–1059.*) Retrograde menstruation is currently believed to be the major cause of endometriosis. Supporting this belief are the following findings: inversion of the uterine cervix into the peritoneal cavity can cause monkeys to develop endometriosis; endometrial tissue is viable outside the uterus; and blood can issue from the ends of the fallopian tubes of some women during menstruation. The fact that endometrial implants can occur in the lung implies that lymphatic or vascular routes of spread of the disease also are possible. Another theory of the etiology of endometriosis entails the conversion of celomic epithelium into glands resembling those of the endometrium. Endometriosis in men, or in women without müllerian structures, is an example of this causative mechanism.

400. The answer is c. *(Speroff, 6/e, pp 441–442.)* Since this patient has other signs of pubertal development which are sex steroid–dependent, we can conclude some ovarian function is present. This excludes such conditions as gonadal dysgenesis and hypothalamic-pituitary failure as possible causes of her primary amenorrhea. Müllerian defects are the only plausible cause, and the diagnostic evaluation in this patient would be directed toward both confirmation of this diagnosis and establishment of the exact nature of the müllerian defect. Müllerian agenesis, also known as Mayer-Rokitansky-Küster-Hauser syndrome, presents as amenorrhea with absence of a vagina. The incidence is approximately 1 in 10,000 female births. The karyotype is 46,XX. There is normal development of breasts, sexual hair, ovaries, tubes, and external genitalia. There are associated skeletal (12%) and urinary tract (33%) anomalies. Treatment generally consists of progressive vaginal dilation or creation of an artificial vagina with split-thickness skin grafts (McIndoe procedure). Testicular feminization, or congenital androgen insensitivity syndrome, is an X-linked recessive disorder with a karyotype of 46,XY. These genetic males have a defective androgen receptor and/or downstream signal transduction mechanism (in the genome), such that the androgenic signal does not have its normal tissue-specific effects. This accounts for 10% of all cases of primary amenorrhea. The patient presents with an absent uterus and blind vaginal canal. However, in these patients the amount of sexual hair is significantly decreased. Although there is a 25% incidence of malignant tumors in these patients, gonadectomy should be deferred until after full development is obtained. In other patients with a Y chromosome, gonadectomy should be performed as early as possible to prevent masculinization. Patients with gonadal dysgenesis present with lack of secondary sexual characteristics.

Patients with Klinefelter syndrome typically have a karyotype of 47,XXY and a male phenotype. Causes of primary amenorrhea in descending order of frequency are gonadal dysgenesis, müllerian agenesis, and testicular feminization. XYY and Turner syndrome often present with menstrual difficulties, but these patients have a uterus.

401. The answer is e. (*Speroff, 6/e, pp 557–567.*) Premenstrual syndrome is a constellation of symptoms that occur in a cyclic pattern, always in the same phase of the menstrual cycle. These symptoms usually occur 7 to 10 days before the onset of menses. Examples of symptoms reported include edema, mood swings, depression, irritability, breast tenderness, increased appetite, and cravings for sweets. The etiology is unclear. Besides the treatments listed in the question, therapy has included oral contraceptives, danazol, bromocriptine, evening primrose oil, and aerobic exercise. Controlled studies have been performed with most of the different treatment regimens with variable, unreproducible, and generally disappointing results that probably are the result of patient heterogeneity because of difficulty in diagnosing this condition. Of all the medications studied, SSRIs have shown the greatest efficacy in PMS treatment.

402. The answer is a. (*Speroff, 6/e, p 581.*) Menorrhagia (excessive but regular menstrual bleeding) is a common problem in women of all ages. Irregular vaginal bleeding is termed metrorrhagia. Preliminary evaluation would include a history, physical examination, pelvic examination, Pap smear, pregnancy test (if applicable), and endometrial biopsy in some patients. Therapeutic alternatives include cyclic low-dose oral contraceptives and progestin therapy for 10 to 14 days on days 14 to 28 of the cycle. Antiprostaglandins (eg., the nonsteroidal anti-inflammatory agents such as ibuprofen, naproxen, etc.) have been shown to significantly decrease menstrual loss. Endometrial biopsy in the second half of the cycle rules out an inadequate luteal phase or anovulatory bleeding. If the bleeding does not resolve with medical therapy, hysteroscopy can be performed to rule out submucous myomas or endometrial polyps. A subserous myoma can occasionally be palpated on pelvic examination or visualized on laparoscopy; however, it is not a cause of dysfunctional uterine bleeding. Hysteroscopy may identify endometrial septa or tubal occlusion, but these are not related to abnormal bleeding.

403. The answer is b. (*Speroff, 6/e, pp 464–469.*) In recent years, the number of women engaged in strenuous recreational activities and competitive sports has significantly increased, resulting in the problem of exercise-induced amenorrhea. Two factors appear to influence the appearance of amenorrhea in these patients: a critical level of body fat appears to be necessary for menstruation; and high energy output and stress appear to act independently in suppressing reproductive function. With vigorous exercise, circulating levels of β-endorphin, β-lipotropin, and adrenocorticotropic hormone (ACTH) are increased. This increase in endogenous opiates might explain the feeling of euphoria that some people get after extensive exercising. Exercise is also associated with an increase in prolactin and growth hormone. There is a suppression of the pulsatile secretion of gonadotropin-releasing hormone (GnRH) with a decrease in gonadotropin release in these patients.

404. The answer is c. (*Speroff, 6/e, pp 605–607.*) Amenorrhea and galactorrhea may be seen when something causes an increase in prolactin secretion or action. The differential diagnosis involves several possible causes. Excessive estrogens, such as with birth control pills, can reduce prolactin-inhibiting factor, thus raising serum prolactin level. Similarly, intensive suckling (during lactation and associated with sexual foreplay) can activate the reflex arc that results in hyperprolactinemia. Many antipsychotic medications, especially the phenothiazines, are also known to have mammotropic properties. Hypothyroidism appears to cause galactorrhea secondary to thyrotropin-releasing hormone (TRH) stimulation of prolactin release. With persistent elevated prolactin levels without obvious cause (e.g., breast feeding), an evaluation for pituitary adenoma becomes necessary.

405. The answer is c. (*Scott, 8/e, pp 615–618. Ransom 1997, pp 570–580.*) The presence of estrogen in a pubertal girl stimulates the formation of secondary sex characteristics, including development of breasts, production of cervical mucus, and vaginal cornification. As estrogen levels increase, menses begins and ovulation is maintained for several decades. Ovarian estrogen production late in puberty is at least in part responsible for termination of the pubertal growth spurt, thereby determining adult height. Decreasing levels of estrogen are associated with lower frequency of ovulation, eventually leading to menopause. Hair growth during puberty is caused by androgens from the adrenal gland and, later, the ovary.

406. The answer is e. (*Speroff, 6/e, pp 392–403.*) These GnRH results and LH pulses are seen in normal puberty. Normal signs of puberty involve breast budding (thelarche, 9.8 years), pubic hair (pubarche, 10.5 years), and menarche (12.8 years). Besides an increase in androgens and a moderate rise in FSH and LH levels, one of the first indications of puberty is an increase in the amplitude and frequency of nocturnal LH pulses. In patients with idiopathic true precocious puberty, the pituitary response to GnRH is identical to that in girls undergoing normal puberty. Iatrogenic sexual precocity (i.e., the accidental ingestion of estrogens), premature thelarche, and ovarian tumors are examples of sexual precocity independent of GnRH, FSH, and LH function.

407–412. The answers are 407-a, 408-d, 409-d, 410-d, 411-d, 412-c. (*Speroff, 6/e, pp 201–237. Adashi, pp 24–40.*) The selection of a primordial follicle to become a dominant follicle with ovulation and development of a corpus luteum is a complex process. Initially, granulosa cells are stimulated by FSH to aromatize androstenedione and testosterone in the granulosa cell to estrone and estradiol. The rise in estradiol exerts a positive feedback on LH. LH receptors are primarily found at this stage in the theca cells, which stimulate production of androgen, which in turn serves as the substrate for further estrogen production. Increasing estrogen and FSH levels induce the appearance of LH receptors on granulosa cells, increase the number of FSH receptors on these granulosa cells, and stimulate granulosa cell proliferation. These cellular actions cause the follicle to grow into a mature, antral preovulatory follicle. After ovulation the follicle becomes a successful corpus luteum under the action of LH.

413. The answer is b. (*Speroff, 6/e, pp 1078–1079.*) Because of the variability in semen specimens from the same person, preferably three specimens should be evaluated over the course of an investigation for infertility. A normal semen analysis will demonstrate at least 20 million sperm per milliliter, over 60% of the sperm with a normal shape, a volume of between 2 and 6 mL, and at least 50% of the sperm with progressive forward motility.

414–418. The answers are 414-a, 415-b, 416-c, 417-e, 418-f. (*Rock, 8/e, pp 550–555. Speroff, 6/e, pp 1025–1027.*) Hysterosalpingography is an important tool in the evaluation of infertility. It provides information regarding the shape of the uterine cavity and the patency of the tubes.

Tubal factors, many of which follow from sexually transmitted diseases, are an important cause of infertility. The figure in question 414 displays bilateral hydrosalpinx and clubbing of the tubes with no evidence of any spillage into the peritoneal cavity. The uterine cavity in this HSG is normal. In the figure in question 408, there is unilateral hydrosalpinx and evidence of adhesions within the uterine cavity consistent with Asherman syndrome. There is no filling of the other tube. In the figure in question 416, one tube fills and has unilateral hydrosalpinx; the other shows loculation and minimal fluid accumulation. The uterine cavity here is normal, in contrast to the cavity shown in question 415. The figure in question 417 shows salpingitis isthmica nodosa in which there is a characteristic "salt-and-pepper" pattern to tubal filling and evidence of a diverticulum of the tube on one side. The figure in question 418 shows normal filling and spillage of contrast media. This is a normal hysterosalpingogram. None of the figures show bilateral proximal occlusion.

419–423. The answers are 419-e, 420-c, 421-b, 422-d, 423-a.
(Adashi, pp 1898–1913. Speroff, 6/e, pp 1013–1037.) The diagnostic evaluation of an infertile couple should be thorough and completed as rapidly as possible. The primary diagnostic steps in the workup of the infertile couple include (1) documentation of ovulation by measurement of basal body temperature (BBT) or mid-luteal phase serum progesterone; (2) semen analysis; (3) postcoital test; (4) hysterosalpingogram; and (5) endometrial biopsy. Women should record their BBT for evidence of ovulation. In addition, serial serum progesterone levels may be helpful to confirm ovulation. Serum progesterone values should be obtained 7 days after ovulation and may also be helpful in evaluating inadequate luteal phase. An endometrial biopsy may also provide valuable information regarding the status of the luteal phase. The biopsy is obtained 12 days after the thermogenic shift, or 2 to 3 days before the expected onset of menses, on about day 26 of a 28-day cycle. A postcoital test is an in vivo test that evaluates the interaction of sperm and cervical mucus. It is performed during the periovulatory period up to 12 h after coitus. The cervical mucus is obtained, and its quantity and quality as well as its interaction with the sperm are evaluated. The hysterosalpingogram is performed in the midfollicular phase in order to evaluate the fallopian tubes and the contour of the uterine cavity; it should not be done while the patient is menstruating or after ovulation has occurred. Although

gonadotropin levels are not routinely evaluated, they should be obtained in the early follicular phase when testing is indicated, e.g., in cases where there is a history of oligoovulation.

424–428. The answers are 424-a, 425-c, 426-b, 427-d, 428-d. *(Speroff, 6/e, pp 39–43. Adashi, pp 1555–1569.)* Testosterone reaching a target organ is converted to dihydrotestosterone by 5α-reductase, an enzyme in the androgen receptor of target organs and tissues such as hair follicles, sebaceous glands, etc. Adenylcyclase, an intracellular enzyme activated by the presence of LH, catalyzes the formation of cyclic adenosine 5′-monophosphate (AMP), which then activates other intracellular enzyme reactions. The enzyme 17β-hydroxysteroid dehydrogenase is found primarily in the testis but also in the adrenal gland; it converts androstenedione to testosterone by reducing the 17 position. The conversion of cholesterol into steroid hormones begins with hydroxylation at the 30 position, followed by cleavage of the six-carbon side chain (carbons 22 to 27); both reactions, which result in production of pregnenolone, are catalyzed by cholesterol desmolase. Congenital deficiencies of this enzyme can cause the adrenal glands to fill with cholesterol and become greatly enlarged; affected infants, some of whom may be phenotypic females but genotypic males, have a poor prognosis. Do not confuse this enzyme with 21-hydroxylase, an enzyme involved in the production of mineralocorticoids and glucocorticoids. Complete forms of 21-hydroxylase deficiency congenital adrenal hyperplasia (CAH) are fatal during the neonatal period unless the salt-wasting syndrome is identified and corrected. Patients with late-onset CAH (LOCAH, or incomplete 21-hydroxylase deficiency) are phenotypically similar to patients with polycystic ovarian syndrome (PCOS), and at times can only be distinguished from them using gonadotropin and androgen tests. For example, in LOCAH 17-hydroxyprogesterone and DHAS levels are elevated and gonadotropins are normal, while in PCOS gonadotropins are elevated and these steroids are typically normal. LOCAH is a common cause of menstrual irregularity and mild hirsutism, usually presenting in the early third decade.

BENIGN AND MALIGNANT NEOPLASMS

Questions

DIRECTIONS: Each item below contains a question or incomplete statement followed by suggested responses. Select the **one best** response to each question.

429. A patient is diagnosed with carcinoma of the breast. The most important prognostic factor in the treatment of this disease is

a. Age at diagnosis
b. Size of tumor
c. Axillary metastases
d. Estrogen receptors on the tumor
e. Progesterone receptors on the tumor

430. Transvaginal ultrasound with Doppler color flow imaging is used to detect malignant ovarian tumors on the basis of the

a. Different temperature of tumor tissue
b. Ultrasonographic pattern of ovarian tumors
c. Increased blood flow of ovarian arteries
d. Neovascularity of tumor blood supply
e. Discordance of ovarian artery blood supply between left to right ovaries

431. Of the following, the most promising technique for ovarian cancer screening in otherwise low-risk women is

a. Transabdominal ultrasound
b. Transvaginal ultrasound
c. Detection of P-53
d. Detection of P-32
e. Detection of carcinoembryonic antigen (CEA)

432. A 21-year-old woman presents with left lower quadrant pain. An anterior 7-cm firm adnexal cyst is palpated. Ultrasound confirms a complex left adnexal mass with solid components that appear to contain bone and teeth. What percentage of these tumors are bilateral?

a. Less than 1%
b. 2% to 3%
c. 10% to 15%
d. 50%
e. Greater than 75%

433. A 54-year-old woman undergoes a laparotomy because of a pelvic mass. At exploratory laparotomy, a unilateral ovarian neoplasm is discovered that is accompanied by a large omental metastasis. Frozen section diagnosis confirms metastatic serous cystadenocarcinoma. The most appropriate intraoperative course of action is

a. Excision of the omental metastasis and ovarian cystectomy
b. Omentectomy and ovarian cystectomy
c. Excision of the omental metastasis and unilateral oophorectomy
d. Omentectomy and bilateral salpingo-oophorectomy
e. Omentectomy, total abdominal hysterectomy, and bilateral salpingo-oophorectomy

434. The primary mode of treatment for endometrial carcinoma confined to the uterine corpus is

a. External beam radiation
b. Intracavitary radium
c. Hysterectomy
d. Chemotherapy
e. Progestin therapy

435. Fractional dilation and curettage reveals endometrial carcinoma involving the cervix. This finding is

a. Of no prognostic significance
b. Of some prognostic significance, but does not require change in management
c. Significant only if the cervical tumor is clinically obvious
d. Significant even if the disease is present only microscopically
e. A contraindication for hysterectomy

436. Ovarian neoplasms most commonly arise from

a. Celomic epithelium
b. Nonspecific mesenchyme
c. Specialized gonadal stroma
d. Primitive germ cells
e. Connective tissue elements within the ovary

437. The most common presentation of primary vaginal cancer is

a. Abnormal bleeding or discharge
b. Pruritus
c. Pelvic pain
d. Lymphadenopathy or lymphedema
e. Symptoms from distant metastases

438. A 58-year-old woman is seen for evaluation of a swelling in her right vulva. She has also noted pain in this area when walking and during coitus. At the time of pelvic examination, a mildly tender, fluctuant mass is noted just outside the introitus in the right vulva in the region of the Bartholin's gland. What is the most appropriate treatment?

a. Marsupialization
b. Administration of antibiotics
c. Surgical excision
d. Incision and drainage
e. Observation

439. A 51-year-old woman is diagnosed with invasive cervical carcinoma by cone biopsy. Pelvic examination and rectal vaginal examination reveal the parametrium to be free of disease, but the upper portion of the vagina is involved with tumor. Intravenous pyelography (IVP) and sigmoidoscopy are negative, but a computed tomography (CT) scan of the abdomen and pelvis shows grossly enlarged pelvic and periaortic nodes. This patient is classified as stage

a. IIa
b. IIb
c. IIIa
d. IIIb
e. IV

Items 440–441

A 35-year-old G3, P3 patient with a pap smear showing high-grade squamous intraepithelial lesion of the cervix (CIN III) has an inadequate colposcopy. Cone biopsy shows squamous cell cancer that has invaded only 1 mm beyond the basement membrane. There are no confluent tongues of tumor, and there is no evidence of lymphatic or vascular invasion. The margins of the cone biopsy specimen are free of disease.

440. How would you classify or stage this patient's disease?

a. Carcinoma of low malignant potential
b. Microinvasive cancer
c. Atypical squamous cells of undetermined significance
d. Carcinoma in situ
e. Invasive cancer, stage IA

441. Of the following, appropriate therapy for this lesion is

a. External beam radiation therapy
b. Implantation of radioactive cesium
c. Simple hysterectomy
d. Simple hysterectomy with pelvic lymphadenectomy
e. Radical hysterectomy

442. Borderline malignant epithelial neoplasms of the ovary are defined as tumors with

a. Only high degrees of mitotic activity
b. Epithelial stratification of two to three layers and cellular atypicality
c. Leukocytic infiltration
d. Only a single focus of malignant degeneration in the neoplasm
e. Higher than usual response to radiation therapy

443. Women who have ovarian carcinoma most commonly present with which of the following symptoms?

a. Vaginal bleeding and anorexia
b. Weight loss and dyspareunia
c. Nausea and vaginal discharge
d. Constipation and frequent urination
e. Abdominal distention and pain

444. The class of chemotherapeutic agents that is most effective in the management of women who have recurrent endometrial carcinoma is

a. Antimetabolites
b. Hormones
c. Alkylating agents
d. Vinca alkaloids
e. Antibiotics

445. Which of the following is a true statement regarding the presence of malignant cells within the peritoneum of patients with endometrial carcinoma?

a. Positive peritoneal washings are of no clinical value
b. Peritoneal washings reveal malignant cells in approximately 15% of stage I tumors
c. The risk of recurrence is not increased with positive peritoneal washings
d. Intraperitoneal P-32 is ineffective when malignant washings are positive
e. The presence of other good prognostic factors negates the significance of malignant washings

446. Women who have endometrial carcinoma most frequently present with which of the following symptoms?

a. Bloating
b. Weight loss
c. Postmenopausal bleeding
d. Vaginal discharge
e. Hemoptysis

447. A woman is found to have a unilateral, invasive vulvar carcinoma that is 2 cm in diameter but not associated with evidence of lymph node spread. Initial management should consist of

a. Chemotherapy
b. Radiation therapy
c. Simple vulvectomy
d. Radical vulvectomy
e. Radical vulvectomy and bilateral inguinal lymphadenectomy

448. Which of the following best describes the usual presentation of invasive cervical carcinoma?

a. Watery, blood-tinged vaginal discharge
b. Significant hemorrhage
c. Pelvic pain
d. Renal failure from ureteral obstruction in the pelvis
e. Evidence of distant metastases

449. A patient is receiving external beam radiation for treatment of metastatic endometrial cancer. The treatment field includes the entire pelvis. Which of the following tissues within this radiation field is the most radiosensitive?

a. Vagina
b. Ovary
c. Rectovaginal septum
d. Bladder
e. Rectum

450. An intravenous pyelogram (IVP) showing hydronephrosis in the workup of a patient with cervical cancer otherwise confined to a cervix of normal size would indicate stage

a. I
b. II
c. III
d. IV
e. V

451. Paget's disease is most often found at which sites?

a. Vulva or nipple
b. Vulva or neck
c. Nipple or axilla
d. Axilla or groin
e. Anywhere on the body

452. Of the following, the most significant risk factor for developing breast cancer is

a. Sclerosing adenosis
b. Ductal ectasia
c. Atypical lobular hyperplasia
d. Fibroadenoma
e. Intraductal papilloma

453. The most common type of breast cancer is

a. Paget's disease of the breast
b. Sarcoma
c. Infiltrating ductal carcinoma
d. Intraductal papilloma
e. Inflammatory carcinoma

454. If a point 2.5 cm from a source of radiation receives a dose of 1000 rads, a point 5 cm from the source of radiation will receive a dose of

a. 250 rads
b. 500 rads
c. 1000 rads
d. 2000 rads
e. 4000 rads

455. Factors associated with poor prognosis in metastatic gestational trophoblastic neoplasia (GTN) include

a. Ectopic pregnancy 3 mo earlier
b. Spontaneous abortion 2 mo previously
c. Pretreatment human chorionic gonadotropin (hCG) titer <10,000 mIU/mL
d. Lung metastasis on chest x-ray
e. Prior chemotherapy

456. Proto-oncogenes are defined as

a. Genes that control the immune system
b. Viral oncogenes that have tumor-transforming capabilities
c. Genes involved in protection from tumors
d. Genes with tumor-transforming capabilities
e. Genes that organize embryonic ovary formation

457. A pregnant 35-year-old patient is at highest risk for the concurrent development of which of the following malignancies?

a. Cervix
b. Ovary
c. Breast
d. Vagina
e. Colon

458. Which of the following are known causes of an abnormal Pap smear?

a. Flat condyloma
b. Treated atrophic changes
c. Vaginitis
d. Previous inflammatory Pap smear
e. Previous chemotherapy for leukemia

459. A 27-year-old patient previously treated with external beam radiation for stage Ib cervical cancer has a central recurrence two years later. A curative surgical procedure is contemplated in which the uterus, both adnexa, and the rectum and bladder will be removed, diverting the fecal stream with a colostomy and the urinary stream with an ileal conduit. What is this procedure called?

a. Radical hysterectomy
b. Supraradical hysterectomy
c. Hemiexenteration
d. Total pelvic exenteration
e. Radical exenteration

460. Stage Ib cervical cancer is diagnosed in a young woman who wishes to retain her ability to have sexual intercourse. Your consultant has therefore recommended a radical hysterectomy. Assuming that the cancer is confined to the cervix and that intraoperative biopsies are negative, which of the following structures would not be removed during the radical hysterectomy?

a. Uterosacral and uterovesical ligaments
b. Pelvic nodes
c. The entire parametrium on both sides of the cervix
d. Both ovaries
e. Upper third of the vagina

461. Adoption of the Bethesda System for Pap smear classifications has resulted in

a. A lower proportion of specimens termed inadequate
b. The use of the term *atypical* for all cytologic abnormalities of clinical significance
c. A cost to the U.S. health care system of $1 billion per year
d. Acceptance of specimens as adequate in the absence of endocervical cells
e. A reduction in the percentage of cases termed atypical

462. The risk of breast cancer is increased by

a. Teenage pregnancy
b. Multiparity
c. Late menarche
d. First pregnancy after age 30
e. Lactation

463. A 24-year-old woman presents with new-onset right lower quadrant pain, and you palpate an enlarged, tender right adnexa. Which of the following sonographic characteristics of the cyst in this patient suggests the need for surgical exploration now instead of observation for one menstrual cycle?

a. Lack of ascites
b. Unilocularity
c. Papillary vegetation
d. 5 cm diameter
e. Demonstration of arterial and venous flow by Doppler imaging

464. Which of the following genital tract abnormalities are found with a higher frequency in women who have been exposed in utero to diethylstilbestrol (DES)?

a. Imperforate hymen
b. Lichen sclerosus
c. Bicornuate uterus
d. Cockscomb cervix
e. Longitudinal vaginal septum

465. Which of the following ovarian tumors is correctly matched with its neoplastic cell type?

	Ovarian Tumor	Neoplastic Cell Type
(A)	Dysgerminoma	Germ cell
(B)	Granulosa cell tumor	Germ cell
(C)	Choriocarcinoma	Celomic epithelium
(D)	Endodermal sinus tumor	Stroma
(E)	Embryonal carcinoma	Transitional epithelium

466. Endodermal sinus tumors are identified by secretion of which of the following tumor markers?

a. Human chorionic gonadotropin (hCG)
b. Carcinoembryonic antigen (CEA)
c. α-fetoprotein (AFP)
d. CA-125
e. BRCA1

467. Which of the following is a homologous sarcoma of the uterus?

a. Rhabdomyosarcoma
b. Leiomyosarcoma
c. Osteosarcoma
d. Chondrosarcoma
e. Liposarcoma

468. A postmenopausal woman receives 3000 rads of pelvic radiation postoperatively after total abdominal hysterectomy with bilateral salpingo-oophorectomy for endometrial adenocarcinoma. Assuming that the field of radiation includes all of the organs below, which organ is most susceptible to radiation injury?

a. Kidney
b. Bladder
c. Vaginal mucosa
d. Bowel
e. Rectum

469. Factors that improve the prognosis for endometrial carcinoma include

a. Grade III histology
b. Younger age
c. Clear cell histologic type
d. Black race
e. Papillary serous histologic type

470. A 70-year-old woman presents for evaluation of a pruritic lesion on the vulva. Examination shows a white, friable lesion on the right labia majora that is 3 cm in diameter, no other suspicious areas are noted. Biopsy of the lesion confirms squamous cell carcinoma. In this patient, lymphatic drainage characteristically is first to the

a. External iliac lymph nodes
b. Superficial inguinal lymph nodes
c. Deep femoral lymph nodes
d. Periaortic nodes
e. Internal iliac nodes

471. A 7-year-old girl is seen by her pediatrician for left lower quadrant pain. You are consulted because an ovarian neoplasm is identified by ultrasound. Of the following, the most common ovarian tumor in this type of patient is

a. Germ cell
b. Papillary serous epithelial
c. Fibrosarcoma
d. Brenner tumor
e. Sarcoma botyroides

472. Epithelial ovarian tumors of low potential malignancy (borderline malignancies) can be described by which of the following statements?

a. They represent nearly half of all epithelial ovarian tumors
b. Ten-year survival rates of stage I tumors are about 50%
c. They are occasionally associated with late recurrences and death
d. They never metastasize within the peritoneal cavity
e. They are associated with destructive infiltration of the ovarian stroma

473. A 41-year-old woman undergoes exploratory laparotomy for a persistent adnexal mass. Frozen section diagnosis is serous carcinoma. Assuming that the other ovary is grossly normal, what is the likelihood that the contralateral ovary is involved in this malignancy?

a. 5%
b. 15%
c. 33%
d. 50%
e. 75%

474. Meigs syndrome is not associated with which of the following tumors?

a. Brenner tumor
b. Ovarian fibroma
c. Thecoma
d. Subserous myoma
e. Granulosa cell tumor

475. Which characteristic of mucinous ovarian carcinoma listed below does not contribute to its higher 5-year survival compared to serous carcinoma of the ovary?

a. Earlier stage at diagnosis
b. Higher rate of unilaterality
c. Small size
d. Good differentiation

476. Relatively good prognosis is found for ovarian epithelial carcinoma with

a. Advanced stage
b. Large volume
c. Well-differentiated histologic appearance
d. Presence of ascites

477. Endometrial carcinoma may contain additional cell types in addition to the malignant glandular elements. Experience with tumors containing these additional cell types suggests that

a. Poor prognosis is because of squamous cell hypertrophy
b. Poorly differentiated adenosquamous cancers have a poor prognosis
c. Adenoacanthomas have a poor prognosis
d. Clear cell carcinomas have a good prognosis
e. Adenosquamous tumors occur more often in young women

478. Which of the following factors increases the risk for endometrial carcinoma?

a. Premature menopause
b. Combination (estrogen and progestogen) hormone replacement therapy
c. Diabetes
d. Low body mass index
e. Multiparity

479. The spread of endometrial adenocarcinoma from the uterine corpus can be described by which of the following statements?

a. Distant organs, such as the liver, are frequently involved
b. Dissemination is mostly by way of the lymphatics
c. The tumor resembles cervical carcinoma in its frequency of dissemination
d. Direct extension is an uncommon route of dissemination
e. The ovaries are the most common metastatic site

480. Considering all stages and degrees of differentiation, the overall five-year survival rate for women diagnosed with adenocarcinoma of the endometrium is approximately

a. 10%
b. 25%
c. 50%
d. 75%
e. 95%

481. Carcinoma of the fallopian tube can be described by which of the following statements?

a. It accounts for approximately 10% of primary malignancies of the genital tract
b. Bilateral involvement occurs in approximately 50% of affected patients
c. Its microscopic appearance can be papillary or papillary-alveolar
d. It is considered only mildly malignant and is associated with a good 5-year survival rate
e. Its diagnosis commonly follows an abnormal Pap smear

482. A postmenopausal woman presents with pruritic white lesions on the vulva. Punch biopsy of a representative area is obtained. Which of the following histologic findings is consistent with the diagnosis of lichen sclerosus from this biopsy?

a. Blunting or loss of the rete pegs
b. Presence of a thickened keratin layer
c. Acute inflammatory infiltration
d. Increase in the number of cellular layers in the epidermis
e. Presence of mitotic figures

483. Which of the following statements characterizes epidermoid carcinoma of the vulva?

a. It arises from the Bartholin's glands
b. It is associated with an increased incidence of epidermoid carcinoma of the endocervix
c. It is seen less frequently than adenocarcinoma
d. It tends to develop in women who are younger than those affected by adenocarcinoma
e. It tends to be more advanced than adenocarcinoma when diagnosed

484. Chemotherapeutic agents that are cell cycle specific include

a. Vincristine
b. Chlorambucil
c. Melphalan
d. Cyclophosphamide (Cytoxan)
e. Thiotepa

DIRECTIONS: Each group of questions below consists of lettered options followed by numbered items. For each numbered item, select the appropriate lettered option(s). Each lettered option may be used once, more than once, or not at all. **Choose exactly the number of options indicated following each item.**

Items 485–486

Match each description with the correct condition.

a. Infection by human papillomavirus (HPV) type 11
b. Infection by HPV type 16
c. Infection by HPV type 18
d. Lichen sclerosus
e. Hyperplastic dystrophy

485. Considered premalignant **(SELECT 3 CONDITIONS)**

486. Associated with benign condyloma **(SELECT 1 CONDITION)**

Items 487–492

For each description that follows, select the ovarian tumor with which it is most likely to be associated.

a. Granulosa tumor
b. Sertoli-Leydig cell tumor
c. Immature teratoma
d. Gonadoblastoma
e. Krukenberg tumor

487. Frequently associated with virilization **(SELECT 1 TUMOR)**

488. Frequently associated with endometrial carcinoma **(SELECT 1 TUMOR)**

489. Tends to recur more than 5 years following the original diagnosis **(SELECT 1 TUMOR)**

490. Calcifications present on pelvic radiographs **(SELECT 1 TUMOR)**

491. Correlation between malignant potential and the amount of embryogenic tissue **(SELECT 1 TUMOR)**

492. Large number of signet ring adenocarcinoma cells **(SELECT 1 TUMOR)**

Items 493–498

Match the chemotherapeutic agents and common side effects.

a. Hemorrhagic cystitis
b. Renal failure
c. Tympanic membrane fibrosis
d. Necrotizing enterocolitis
e. Pulmonary fibrosis
f. Pancreatic failure
g. Ocular degeneration
h. Cardiac toxicity
i. Peripheral neuropathy
j. Bone marrow depression

493. Cyclophosphamide
(SELECT 1 SIDE EFFECT)

494. Cisplatin **(SELECT 1 SIDE EFFECT)**

495. Taxol **(SELECT 1 SIDE EFFECT)**

496. Bleomycin **(SELECT 1 SIDE EFFECT)**

497. Doxorubicin **(SELECT 1 SIDE EFFECT)**

498. Vincristine **(SELECT 1 SIDE EFFECT)**

Items 499–505

Match each figure with the correct description **(SELECT 1 DE-SCRIPTION)**.

a. Well-differentiated adenocarcinoma of the endometrium (FIGO I/III)
b. Proliferative endometrium
c. Choriocarcinoma
d. Late secretory endometrium
e. Mixed müllerian endometrial cancer
f. Mature cystic teratoma
g. Clear cell cancer of the endometrium

499

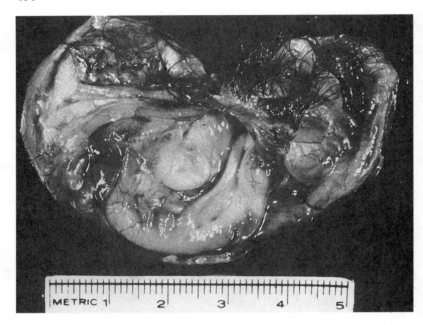

500

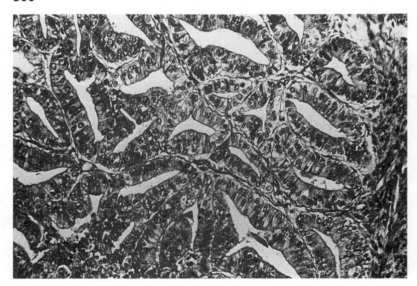

501

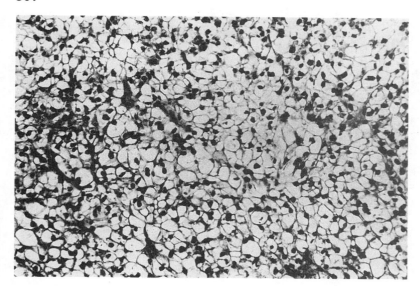

502

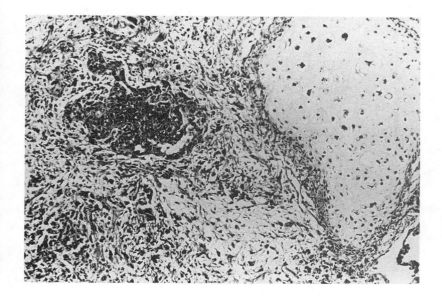

503

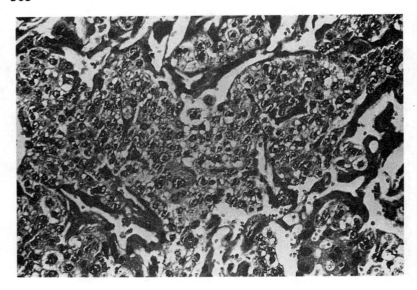

504

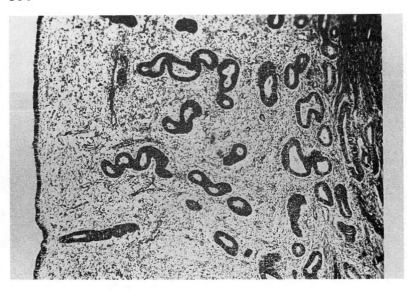

505

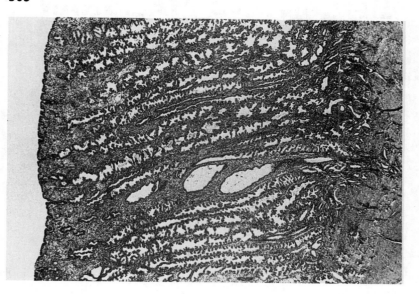

BENIGN AND MALIGNANT NEOPLASMS

Answers

429. The answer is c. *(Hoskins, 2/e, pp 1094–1095.)* Recognition of the high risk associated with axillary metastases for early death and poor five-year survival has led to the use of postsurgical adjuvant chemotherapy in these patients. Patients who have estrogen- or progesterone-receptive tumors (i.e., receptor present or receptor positive) are particular candidates for this adjuvant therapy, as 60% of estrogen-positive tumors will respond to hormonal therapy. Age and size of the tumor are certainly factors of importance, but they are secondary in importance to the presence or absence of axillary metastases.

430. The answer is d. *(Hoskins, 2/e, p 937.)* Transvaginal ultrasound aided by Doppler color flow techniques is improving the ability to detect ovarian tumors at early stages. The neovascularity of tumor tissue is the basis upon which diagnosis can be made by observing ectopic blood flow patterns. There are no characteristic vascular patterns found in early tumors, nor is there a temperature difference. Differences of blood flow from one side to the other are very unreliable and certainly not generally useful. The sensitivity and specificity of screening by transvaginal ultrasound is not yet proven.

431. The answer is b. *(DiSaia, 5/e, pp 611–612.)* Screening for ovarian cancer in the general population is highly controversial and is not believed to be routinely cost effective. Established biochemical markers such as CA-125, CEA, and P-32 seem to be of relatively little significance, while P-53, a new experimental marker, may be somewhat more promising. All are much better suited to assessment of risk and/or presence of recurrence in patients already diagnosed with ovarian cancer after they have been treated. Ultrasound, particularly with Doppler color flow imaging to look for enhanced blood flow, appears to be much more promising. The transvaginal approach allows for closer placement of the transducer and, therefore, higher resolution and subsequent sensitivity compared with the transabdominal route. Multimodal screening using ultrasound coupled with serum markers may further improve the accuracy of screening in patients.

432. The answer is c. *(Hoskins, 2/e, p 987.)* Benign cystic teratomas are the most common germ cell tumors and account for about 20% to 25% of all ovarian neoplasms. They occur primarily during the reproductive years but may also occur in postmenopausal women and in children. Dermoids are usually unilateral, but 10% to 15% are bilateral. Usually the tumors are asymptomatic, but they can cause severe pain if there is torsion or if the sebaceous material perforates, spills, and creates a reactive peritonitis.

433. The answer is e. *(Hoskins, 2/e, pp 940–944.)* The survival of women who have ovarian carcinoma varies inversely with the amount of residual tumor left after the initial surgery. At the time of laparotomy, a maximum effort should be made to determine the sites of tumor spread and to excise all resectable tumor. Although the uterus and ovaries may appear grossly normal, there is a relatively high incidence of occult metastases to these organs; for this reason, they should be removed during the initial surgery. Ovarian cancer metastasizes outside the peritoneum via the pelvic or paraaortic lymphatics, and from there into the thorax and the remainder of the body.

434. The answer is c. *(Hoskins, 2/e, pp 1122–1124.)* Hysterectomy (actually simple hysterectomy with bilateral salpingo-oophorectomy) is the primary mode of treatment for women who have endometrial carcinoma confined to the uterine corpus. Because this is primarily a disease of the postmenopausal woman, concerns regarding removal of the ovaries that would be a factor in a woman of reproductive age generally do not concern these patients. External beam and intracavity radiation have been employed to help reduce central and pelvic recurrences of the cancer. Progestin therapy is used routinely as primary treatment for women who have advanced disease or recurrent carcinoma, and chemotherapy is used for patients whose tumors have failed to respond to other forms of therapy.

435. The answer is d. *(Hoskins, 2/e, pp 1122–1124.)* Endometrial carcinoma involving the cervix is significant even if present only as microscopic disease. The lymphatic drainage of the uterine corpus is primarily by way of the lymphatics that follow the ovarian vessels, i.e., to the renal vein on the left and the inferior vena cava on the right. Because involvement of the cervix allows the cancer to metastasize via the parametrial lymphatics, the 5-year survival rate is reduced (regardless of the volume of tumor present) and intense radiation treatment is required. Often this is given as adjuvant postoperative radiotherapy; consequently, hysterectomy need not be excluded from the management program.

436. The answer is a. *(Hoskins, 2/e, pp 460–461.)* Ovarian neoplasms arise more commonly from celomic epithelium than from any other source. Many tumors of this group include epithelium that histologically resembles endocervical, endometrial, or fallopian tube epithelium (giving rise, respectively, to mucinous, endometrioid, and serous carcinomas). Other, less common ovarian tumors of celomic epithelial origin include mesonephroid carcinoma, Brenner tumors, mixed mesodermal tumors, and carcinosarcomas. Epithelial tumors frequently contain mixed cell types; categorization of these tumors is according to the cell type that predominates.

437. The answer is a. *(Hoskins, 2/e, pp 755–766.)* Primary vaginal cancers are rare, constituting less than 2% of all gynecologic malignancies. They are histologically usually classified as squamous cell carcinomas and, present in women over the age of 50 years. Frequently there is a delay in the diagnosis of this carcinoma because of its rarity as well as a lack of association of the symptoms with the disease. The most common symptom is abnormal bleeding or discharge. Both surgery and radiation therapy have been effective; however, radiation therapy has been the most frequent mode of treatment in recent years.

438. The answer is c. *(Hoskins, 2/e, p 728.)* Although rare, adenocarcinoma of Bartholin's gland must be excluded in women over 40 years of age who present with a cystic or solid mass in this area. The appropriate treatment in these cases is surgical excision of the Bartholin's gland to allow for a careful pathologic examination. In cases of abscess formation, both marsupialization of the sac and incision with drainage as well as appropriate antibiotics are accepted modes of therapy. In the case of the asymptomatic Bartholin's cyst, no treatment is necessary.

439. The answer is a. (*Hoskins, 2/e, pp 827–828.*) Cervical cancer is still staged clinically. Physical examination, routine x-rays, barium enema, colposcopy, cystoscopy, proctosigmoidoscopy, and IVP are used to stage the disease. CT scan results, while clinically useful, are not used to stage the disease. Stage I disease is limited to the cervix. Stage Ia disease is preclinical (i.e., microscopic), while stage Ib denotes macroscopic disease. Stage II involves the vagina, but not the lower one-third, or infiltrates the parametrium, but not out to the pelvic sidewall. IIa denotes vaginal but not parametrial extension, while IIb denotes parametrial extension. Stage III involves the lower one-third of the vagina or extends to the pelvic sidewall; there is no cancer-free area between the tumor and the pelvic wall. Stage IIIa lesions have not extended to the pelvic wall, but involve the lower one-third of the vagina. Stage IIIb tumors have extension to the pelvic wall, and/or are associated with hydronephrosis or a nonfunctioning kidney caused by tumor. Stage IV is outside the reproductive tract.

440–441. The answers are 440-b, 441-c. (*Hoskins, 2/e, pp 793–794, 802–803.*) Microinvasive carcinoma of the cervix includes lesions within 3 mm of the base of the epithelium, with no confluent tongues or lymphatic or vascular invasion. The overall incidence of metastases in 751 reported cases is 1.2%. Simple hysterectomy is accepted therapy.

442. The answer is b. (*DiSaia, 5/e, pp 270–274.*) Borderline malignant ovarian neoplasms constitute 15% of epithelial ovarian cancers. The 10-year survival is 95%. Histology reveals minimal degrees of epithelial stratification, pleomorphism, atypicality, and mitotic activity. If the disease is unilateral, a salpingo-oophorectomy is adequate following a benign biopsy of the contralateral ovary. For bilateral disease or intraperitoneal spread, more radical surgery is indicated.

443. The answer is e. (*DiSaia, 5/e, p 290.*) Approximately 50% of women who have ovarian cancer present with abdominal distention, and 50% present with abdominal pain. Gastrointestinal symptoms, which occur in about 20% of affected women, are often secondary to the development of ascites or partial bowel obstruction from the tumor. Urinary tract symptoms, caused by the pressure exerted by a rapidly growing mass, and abnormal vaginal bleeding are the initial symptoms of ovarian cancer in only 15% of affected women.

444. The answer is b. *(DiSaia, 5/e, pp 160–164.)* Hormones, especially progestins, have been employed successfully in the treatment of women who have recurrent endometrial carcinoma. In many series, response rates of 30% to 40% have been noted. The most frequently employed agents have been hydroxyprogesterone caproate (Delalutin) and medroxyprogesterone acetate (Provera). Single-agent chemotherapy with nonhormonal agents has produced disappointing responses in patients affected by advanced or recurrent endometrial carcinoma.

445. The answer is b. *(DiSaia, 5/e, p 149.)* Peritoneal washings are positive in approximately 15% of patients with stage I endometrial cancer. Patients with positive cytology have a three- to fourfold higher risk of recurrence. The presence of malignant peritoneal washings negates other good prognostic factors. Intraperitoneal P-32 has been efficacious in decreasing recurrences in patients with positive washings.

446. The answer is c. *(DiSaia, 5/e, pp 137–142.)* Postmenopausal bleeding is the most common presenting symptom of women who have endometrial carcinoma. Because this warning signal is present even in the earliest stage of the disease, early diagnosis and treatment are possible and likely. In fact, approximately 70% of affected women have stage I disease when they first seek treatment.

447. The answer is e. *(DiSaia, 5/e, pp 153–160.)* Women who have invasive vulvar carcinoma usually are treated surgically. If the lesion is unilateral, is not associated with fixed or ulcerated inguinal lymph nodes, and does not involve the urethra, vagina, anus, or rectum, then treatment usually consists of radical vulvectomy and bilateral inguinal lymphadenectomy. If inguinal lymph nodes show evidence of metastatic disease, bilateral pelvic lymphadenectomy is usually performed. Radiation therapy, though not a routine part of the management of women who have early vulvar carcinoma, is employed (as an alternative to pelvic exenteration with radical vulvectomy) in the treatment of women who have local, advanced carcinoma.

448. The answer is a. *(DiSaia, 5/e, pp 89–91.)* Cervical cancer frequently presents with a watery discharge and postcoital spotting. Surgical staging by the Gynecologic Oncology Group has revealed periaortic node involvement in 5.6% of stage I lesions. Five-year survival rates of approximately 90% are achieved with either surgery or radiation for early-stage disease. Both for initial therapy and recurrent carcinoma, chemotherapy is not as good as the other two treatment modalities; intraarterial chemotherapy administration has not improved this poor response to chemotherapy.

449. The answer is b. *(DiSaia, 5/e, pp 619–622.)* Different tissues tolerate different doses of radiation, but the ovaries are by far the most radiosensitive. They tolerate up to 2,500 rads, while the other tissues listed tolerate between 5,000 and 20,000 rads. Acute evidence of excessive radiation exposure includes tissue necrosis and inflammation, resulting in enteritis, cystitis, vulvitis, proctosigmoiditis, and possible bone marrow suppression. Chronic effects of excessive radiation exposure are manifest months to years after therapy, and include vasculitis, fibrosis, and deficient cellular regrowth; these can result in proctitis, cystitis, fistulas, scarring, and stenosis.

Successful radiation depends upon (1) the greater sensitivity of the cancer cell compared with normal tissue, and (2) the greater ability of normal tissue to repair itself after irradiation. The maximal resistance to ionizing radiation depends on an intact circulation and adequate cellular oxygenation. Resistance also depends upon total dose, number of portions, and time intervals. The relative resistance of normal tissue (cervix and vagina) in cervical cancer allows high surface doses approaching 15,000 to 20,000 rads to be delivered to the tumor with intracavitary devices, and, because of the inverse square law, significantly lower doses of radiation reach the bladder and rectum. The greater the fractionalization (number of portions the total dose is broken into), the better the normal tissue tolerance of that radiation dose; hence 5,000 rads of pelvic radiation is usually given in daily fractions over 5 wk, with approximately 200 rads being administered each day.

450. The answer is c. *(Hoskins, 2/e, pp 790–791.)* By definition, a positive IVP would mean extension to the pelvic sidewall and thus a stage III carcinoma, specifically stage IIIb. Such staging applies even if there is no palpable tumor beyond the cervix. In addition to examination, IVP, cystoscopy, and proctosigmoidoscopy are the diagnostic tests used to stage cervical cancer. However, it is important to understand that while the results of only certain tests are used to stage the cancer, this does not limit the physician from performing any other diagnostic tests (such as CT scans of the abdomen, pelvis, or chest) that in his or her judgment are required for appropriate medical care and decision making.

451. The answer is a. (*Hoskins, 2/e, p 747.*) Paget's cells are most often seen in nests, although single isolated cells can be found. Their large size and pale cytoplasm easily differentiates them from surrounding keratinocytes in the skin. Paget's disease is a clue to the presence of an underlying vulvar adenocarcinoma in approximately 15% of cases, and in about 30% of cases a nongenital adenocarcinoma (most commonly involving the breast, colon, rectum, or upper genital tract) will be present or develop later. Paget's disease commonly occurs in the nipple and vulva, and local recurrences are common. The recommended treatment is wide local excision.

452. The answer is c. (*DiSaia 5/e, pp 390–396.*) The risk for developing breast cancer is increased by a factor of three- to six-fold by the presence of atypical lobular or ductal hyperplasia, especially when cellular atypia is present. While not strictly accurate, these lesions are analogous to severely dysplastic or in situ squamous intraepithelial neoplastic lesions. The other lesions listed are benign. There is considerable debate concerning the impact of the presence of benign breast disease on the subsequent appearance of breast cancer. However, it does appear that the degree and nature of epithelial proliferation (i.e., whether histologically typical or atypical) are important. Fibroadenomas are the most common benign tumors of the breast. In the absence of a suspicious mass, bloody nipple discharge is usually caused by an intraductal papilloma, another benign breast lesion. Neither fibroadenoma or papilloma are associated with a significantly increased incidence of subsequent breast cancer. Ductal ectasia presents with a multicolored, sticky, bilateral discharge in the absence of a defined breast mass. The risk of cancer is also not increased with this lesion. There is also no increase in the risk of breast cancer associated with a diagnosis of sclerosing adenosis, a lesion that simulates carcinoma grossly yet is entirely benign.

453. The answer is c. (*Scott, 8/e, p 641. Mishell, 3/e, pp 374–375.*) Approximately 70% to 80% of malignant breast tumors are infiltrating duct carcinomas. A bloody nipple discharge is most often due to an intraductal papilloma, a benign condition. Carcinoma is detected in up to about 18% of these cases. Breast cysts do not increase the risk for development of breast cancer. Ninety-eight percent of breast masses are found initially by the patient, and 80% of breast cancers have a lump as their first symptom.

454. The answer is a. *(DiSaia, 5/e, pp 619–622.)* The energy from a radiation source varies as the distance it travels from the source varies. This relationship is described by the inverse square law, which states that the energy dose of radiation per unit area decreases proportionately to the square of the distance from the site to the source. Thus, the dose of radiation at 5 cm from a point source is one-fourth (250 rads) the value of the dose at 2.5 cm (1000 rads), since the distance doubles and hence the radiation dose decreases by a factor of $2^2 = 4$.

455. The answer is e. *(DiSaia, 5/e, pp 180–201.)* Gestational trophoblastic disease is a group of diseases including hydatidiform mole, invasive mole, and choriocarcinoma. Gestational trophoblastic neoplasm (GTN) generally refers to invasive moles and choriocarcinoma. GTN is classified as nonmetastatic when there is no evidence of disease outside the uterus and as metastatic when there is any disease outside the uterus. Metastatic GTN is further categorized as good prognosis or poor prognosis. Good prognosis factors include short duration (last pregnancy within 4 mo), low pretreatment hCG titer (<40,000 mIU/mL), no metastasis to brain or liver, and no significant prior chemotherapy. Poor prognosis factors include long duration (last pregnancy >4 mo), high pretreatment hCG titer (>40,000 mIU/mL), brain or liver metastasis, failed prior chemotherapy, and term pregnancy.

456. The answer is d. *(DiSaia, 5/e, pp 581–589.)* The molecular characterization of viral oncogenes led to the discovery of proto-oncogenes, which are in DNA sequences found in the human genome that have tumor-transforming properties. These proto-oncogenes are very similar in structure to viral oncogenes, which have known tumor-transforming capabilities. Proto-oncogenes are intimately involved in the normal functions of cellular growth, differentiation, and proliferation. They are closely related in many respects to known growth factors, which operate through transcriptional mechanisms. Tumor suppressor genes are essentially inhibitory in nature. Removal of tumor suppressor genes allows for unchecked growth and malignant transformation of tumor tissues. Attempts to control tumor growth through biologic therapy and immunotherapy are relatively new techniques that show promise in a number of tumors.

457. The answer is a. (*DiSaia, 5/e, pp 1–16.*) Cervical cancer is a more common gynecologic malignancy in pregnancy than ovarian or breast cancer due to the fact that it is a disease of younger women. Management of cervical intraepithelial lesions is complicated in pregnancy because of increased vascularity of the cervix and because of the concern that manipulation of and trauma to the cervix can compromise continuation of the pregnancy. A traditional cone biopsy is only indicated in the presence of apparent microinvasive disease on a colposcopically directed cervical biopsy. Otherwise, more limited procedures such as shallow coin biopsies are more appropriate. If invasive cancer is diagnosed, the decision to treat immediately or wait until fetal viability depends in part upon the gestational age at which the diagnosis is made and the severity of the disorder. Survival is decreased for malignancies discovered later in pregnancy. Radiation therapy almost always results in spontaneous abortion, in part because the fetus is particularly radiosensitive. Chemotherapy is associated with higher than expected rates of fetal malformations consistent with the antimetabolite effects of agents used. Specific malformations depend upon the agent used and the time in pregnancy at which the exposure occurs.

458. The answer is a. (*DiSaia, 5/e, pp 11–13.*) Any metaplastic process that can produce atypical cells is classified by the Bethesda System as placing the patient at risk. The other conditions named in the question, while not the most likely, must be considered in the evaluation of atypical results. Systemic chemotherapy should not produce atypical cells on Pap smear. Colposcopy would be the next appropriate step with appropriate biopsies and cervical curettage.

459. The answer is d. (*DiSaia, 5/e, pp 93–99.*) Pelvic exenteration has significantly increased the survival rate in recurrent cervical cancer and allowed a quality of life not previously possible. A total pelvic exenteration includes removal of the structures described, with diversion of fecal and urinary streams. Attempts to preserve organs such as the bladder (termed a posterior exenteration, preserving the anterior bladder) or rectum (called an anterior exenteration, preserving the posterior rectum) generally have higher complication rates than a total exenteration and are generally no longer performed. Major improvement in quality of life and electrolyte balance has resulted from the use of an ileal conduit for urinary diversion rather than the earlier technique of tunneling the ureters directly into the transverse colon. Pelvic wall nodes are a contraindication to the surgery, as there is less than a 5% survival rate in such patients.

460. The answer is d. *(DiSaia, 5/e, pp 69–71.)* Radical hysterectomy was popularized by Meigs in the 1940s and has become a very safe procedure in skilled hands. It is most often used as primary treatment for early cervical cancer (stage Ib and IIa), and occasionally as primary treatment for uterine cancer. In either case, there must be no evidence of spread beyond the operative field, as suggested by negative intraoperative frozen section biopsies. The procedure involves excision of the uterus, the upper third of the vagina, the uterosacral and uterovesical ligaments, and all of the parametrium, and pelvic node dissection including the ureteral, obturator, hypogastric, and iliac nodes. Radical hysterectomy thus attempts to preserve the bladder, rectum, and ureters while excising as much as possible of the remaining tissue around the cervix that might be involved in microscopic spread of the disease. Ovarian metastases from cervical cancer are extremely rare. Preservation of the ovaries is generally acceptable, particularly in younger women, unless there is some other reason to consider oophorectomy.

461. The answer is d. *(DiSaia, 5/e, pp 11–13.)* The adoption of the so-called Bethesda System for Pap smear evaluation was the result, in part, of a U.S. federal mandate. Since this system was first proposed in 1988, there has been a gradual transition to its federally mandated use, although there have been some problems along the way. A higher proportion of smears are now termed inadequate because of relatively rigid criteria, although the criteria have been loosened considerably. The term *atypical* applies only to areas of undetermined significance. Abnormalities consistent with a defined process are labeled as such. Endocervical cells do not have to be present for a specimen to be considered adequate, as the risk of missing a significant lesion in their absence is still very small. Finally, the adoption of the Bethesda System has actually led to an increase in the cost of medical care, as the percentage of Pap smears considered abnormal has gone from roughly 5% to 10%. This 5% increase in the number of atypical smears is at an additional cost to the U.S. health care system of approximately $5 billion per year.

462. The answer is d. *(Hoskins, 2/e, p 1084.)* Breast cancer is the most common malady of American women, with 189,000 new cases in 1992 and 44,000 deaths. The incidence increases with age. Risk factors include late pregnancy, nulliparity, and prolonged menstrual life, i.e., early menarche and later menopause. Lactation does not alter incidence, and the effect, if any, of birth control pills is unclear, although probably small.

463. The answer is c. *(DiSaia, 5/e, pp 282–300.)* Approximately 20% of ovarian neoplasms are considered malignant on pathologic examination. However, all must be considered as placing the patient at risk. Given that most ovarian tumors are not found until significant spread has occurred, it is not unreasonable to attempt to operate on such patients as soon as there is a suspicion of tumor. Papillary vegetation, size greater than 10 cm, ascites, possible torsion, or solid lesions are automatic indications for exploratory laparotomy. In a younger woman, a cyst can be followed past one menstrual cycle to determine if it is a follicular cyst, since a follicular cyst should regress after onset of the next menstrual period. If regression does not occur, then surgery is appropriate. Doppler ultrasound imaging allows visualization of arterial and venous flow patterns superimposed upon the image of the structure being examined; arterial and venous flow are expected in a normal ovary.

464. The answer is d. *(Mishell, 3/e, pp 38–39.)* Some women whose mothers were treated with DES during pregnancy show deformities of the upper vagina and cervix. The various deformities include transverse vaginal and cervical ridge, cervical collar, vaginal hood, and cockscomb cervix (an anterior cervical protrusion resembling the comb of a rooster). The upper genital tract can also be affected. The classic deformity of the uterus is a T-shaped configuration with constricting bands in the uterine cavity and a hypoplastic appearance. The lower genital tract abnormalities predispose to cervical and vaginal neoplasia, particularly clear cell adenocarcinoma of the vagina appearing in areas of vaginal adenosis. A T-shaped uterus is associated with increased fetal wastage by spontaneous abortion and premature delivery.

465. The answer is a. (*Hoskins, 2/e, pp 924–932.*) The major classifications of ovarian tumors include epithelial (the most common, including serous and mucinous cystadenocarcinoma), germ cell, and stromal tumors, reflecting the three tissues found within the adult ovary. The germ cell tumors are neoplasms considered to be derived from the primitive germ cells of the embryonic gonad. They consist of dysgerminoma, endodermal sinus tumor, embryonal carcinoma, polyembryoma, choriocarcinoma, gonadoblastoma, and teratoma (dermoid). Granulosa cell tumor is a type of stromal sex cord tumor and often secretes estrogen. Many of the germ cell tumors have important specific characteristics. In dysgerminoma, stroma is often infiltrated with lymphocytes; this is the only germ cell tumor in which the opposite ovary may be involved, and it is acutely sensitive to irradiation. Endodermal sinus tumors may have elevated α-fetoprotein levels, extremely rapid growth, and Schiller-Duval bodies. Choriocarcinoma is associated with elevated hCG levels.

466. The answer is c. (*DiSaia, 5/e, pp 249–250, 355–357.*) Endodermal sinus tumors secrete AFP but not hCG. These tumors occur in females between 13 mo and 45 years of age, with a median age of 19 years at diagnosis. Surgical extirpation of the disease with postoperative chemotherapy is the treatment of choice. hCG is secreted by several tumors, notably choriocarcinoma. CEA and CA-125 are less specific, and are secreted by a variety of begin and malignant disorders. *BRCA1* is a genetic determinant (a DNA sequence, not a circulating secretory product of a tumor) linked to familial syndromes of breast and ovarian cancer.

467. The answer is b. (*Hoskins, 2/e, pp 913–915.*) Uterine sarcomas constitute less than 5% of uterine malignancies. They can be classified by their cell type: homologous sarcomas contain tissue that is normally found in the uterus and heterologous sarcomas contain tissue that is foreign to the uterus. Homologous types include leiomyosarcomas, endometrial stromal sarcomas, and rarely angiosarcomas. Heterologous types include rhabdomyosarcomas, chondrosarcomas, osteosarcomas, and liposarcomas.

468. The answer is a. (*Hoskins, 2/e, pp 314–316.*) The kidney has a tissue tolerance of 2000 to 2300 rads and the liver has a tolerance of 2500 to 3500 rads. The approximate tolerance dose of the bladder, rectum, vaginal mucosa, and bowel is between 6000 and 7000 rads. Beyond these limits, these organs are likely to experience some acute and/or chronic effective of radiation injury.

469. The answer is b. (*Hoskins, 2/e, pp 608–610.*) Studies have shown that younger women with endometrial carcinoma have an improved prognosis. White patients have a higher survival rate than black patients. The histologic type of the endometrial carcinoma is related to prognosis: clear cell carcinoma and papillary serous carcinoma have a worse prognosis than does typical endometrial adenocarcinoma. Tumor grade refers to the degree of anaplasia and differentiation of a tumor, grade III tumors are poorly differentiated, anaplastic tumors with inherently higher malignant potential.

470. The answer is b. (*Hoskins, 2/e, p 720.*) An important feature of the lymphatic drainage of the vulva is the existence of drainage across the midline. The vulva drains first into the superficial inguinal lymph nodes, then into the deep femoral nodes, and finally into the external iliac lymph nodes. The clinical significance of this sequence for patients with carcinoma of the vulva is that the iliac nodes are probably free of the disease if the deep femoral nodes are not involved. Unlike the lymphatic drainage from the rest of the vulva, the drainage from the clitoral region bypasses the superficial inguinal nodes and passes directly to the deep femoral nodes. Thus, while the superficial nodes usually also have metastases when the deep femoral nodes are implicated, it is possible for only the deep nodes to be involved if the carcinoma is in the midline near the clitoris.

471. The answer is b. (*DiSaia, 5/e, p 285.*) The most common ovarian neoplasms in children are of germ cell origin, and about half of these tumors are malignant. Functioning ovarian tumors have been reported to produce precocious puberty in about 2% of affected patients. Epithelial tumors of the ovary, which are quite rare in prepubertal girls, are benign in approximately 90% of all cases; papillary serous cystadenocarcinoma is an example of such a malignant epithelial tumor. Stromal tumors (such as fibrosarcoma) and Brenner tumor are not seen in this age group. Sarcoma botyroides, a tumor seen in children, is a malignancy associated with müllerian structures such as the vagina and uterus, including the uterine cervix.

472. The answer is c. *(Griffiths, pp 172–181.)* Epithelial ovarian tumors of low potential malignancy represent 15% of all epithelial ovarian tumors. Although they do not infiltrate destructively into the ovarian stroma, these borderline malignancies have been associated with late recurrences and death and may metastasize throughout the peritoneal cavity. Histologically, these tumors demonstrate proliferative activity, abnormal mitoses, and nuclear abnormalities. Ten-year survival rates of women who have stage I tumors of low malignant potential have been reported to be 95%; these tumors appear to be safely managed with unilateral oophorectomy.

473. The answer is c. *(Hoskins, 2/e, pp 928–930.)* Serous carcinoma is the most common epithelial tumor of the ovary. On histologic examination, psammoma bodies can be seen in approximately 30% of these tumors. Bilateral involvement characterizes about one-third of all serous carcinomas. Although mesonephroid carcinomas tend to be associated with pelvic endometriosis, a similar association has not been demonstrated for serous carcinomas.

474. The answer is d. *(DiSaia, 5/e, p 268.)* Hydrothorax and ascites are the characteristic features of Meigs syndrome. It is believed that fluid accumulates in the thorax by permeating through diaphragmatic lymphatics. First described in association with ovarian fibromas, Meigs syndrome also can be seen in combination with other ovarian tumors such as Brenner tumors, thecomas, granulosa cell tumors, and other solid ovarian tumors; large subserous uterine myomas, however, are not associated with development of this syndrome.

475. The answer is c. *(Griffiths, pp 172–182.)* Mucinous carcinomas of the ovary are usually diagnosed at an earlier stage than serous carcinomas and tend to be histologically well differentiated. This combination of diagnosis at an early stage (when the tumors frequently are unilateral) and well-differentiated histologic appearance is probably the reason that women who have mucinous carcinoma have a better 5-year survival rate than women affected by serous carcinoma. Mucinous tumors of the ovary, which are less common than serous lesions, usually are lobulated and may grow to enormous proportions.

476. The answer is c. *(Hoskins, 2/e, p 942.)* The extent (or stage) and the volume of a tumor are probably the most important prognostic factors in the management of women with ovarian epithelial carcinoma. However, on a stage-by-stage basis, women who have well-differentiated tumors have better prognoses than women who have poorly differentiated tumors. The presence of ascites or peritoneal washings that are cytologically positive for malignant cells decreases the 5-year survival of affected women.

477. The answer is b. *(Hoskins, 2/e, pp 863–868.)* Recent evidence suggests that adenosquamous carcinoma of the endometrium has a poorer prognosis than either adenocarcinoma or adenoacanthoma of the endometrium. It has yet to be resolved whether the poorer prognosis associated with adenosquamous lesions is due to the population of malignant squamous cells or to the poorly differentiated adenomatous elements, which normally carry a poor prognosis. Adenoacanthoma, which is characterized by benign metaplasia of squamous epithelium, has a prognosis similar to that of other adenocarcinomas of the endometrium. Adenosquamous tumors tend to occur more frequently in older women.

478. The answer is c. *(DiSaia, 5/e, pp 114–116.)* Endometrial carcinoma tends to occur in obese, diabetic women who undergo late-onset menopause and are nulliparous or have low parity. Other factors that may predispose to endometrial carcinoma include hypertension, cancer at other sites (e.g., ovary and breast), and familial history of this malignancy. While unopposed estrogen therapy in menopausal woman increases their risk of endometrial hyperplasia and malignancy, when a progestogen is added (either continuously or cyclically) the incidence of endometrial hyperplasia and neoplasia actually drops below the incidence in women who take no hormone replacement medications.

479. The answer is b. *(Hoskins, 2/e, pp 868–872.)* Although the most common route of dissemination of adenocarcinoma of the uterus is via the lymphatics, this tumor spreads much less often than cervical malignancies and only rarely affects distant organs. Nearby surface structures are affected more frequently, and the cervix, bladder, and rectum can become involved in advanced cases. Direct extension, though not as common as lymphatic dissemination, is also important.

480. The answer is d. *(Griffiths, pp 133–135.)* Endometrial cancer primarily affects women who have passed menopause; on the average, endometrial cancer appears 10 years later than cervical carcinoma. The fact that the frequency of this condition has been increasing recently is certainly due in part to the increased life span of American women. Most studies have revealed a 5-year survival rate of about 75% for women who have endometrial cancer, including all stages, grades, and treatment protocols. This survival rate is highest among all gynecologic malignancies.

481. The answer is c. *(Hoskins, 2/e, pp 1025–1036.)* Because affected women have a low 5-year survival rate, primary tubal carcinoma is thought to be highly malignant; this relationship, however, may be due more to delayed discovery of the tumor than to its malignant potential. Primary tubal carcinoma accounts for only 0.2% to 0.5% of primary malignancies of the genital tract. Microscopically, these tumors present a papillary or papillary-alveolar pattern. Bilateral involvement occurs in about one-fourth of affected women.

482. The answer is a. *(DiSaia, 5/e, pp 41–42.)* Lichen sclerosus was formerly termed lichen sclerosus et atrophicus, but recent studies have concluded that atrophy does not exist. Patients with lichen sclerosus of the vulva tend to be older; they typically present with pruritus, and the lesions are usually white with crinkled skin and well-defined borders. The histologic appearance of lichen sclerosus includes loss of the rete pegs within the dermis, chronic inflammatory infiltrate below the dermis, the development of a homogenous subepithelial layer in the dermis, a decrease in the number of cellular layers, and a decrease in the number of melanocytes. Mechanical trauma has produced bullous areas of lymphedema and lacunae, which are then filled with erythrocytes. Ulcerations and ecchymoses may be seen in these traumatized areas as well. Mitotic figures are rare in lichen sclerosus, and hyperkeratosis is not a feature. While a significant cause of symptoms, lichen sclerosus is not a premalignant lesion. Its importance lies in the fact that it must be distinguished from vulvar squamous cancer.

483. The answer is b. *(Hoskins, 2/e, pp 719–732.)* Epidermoid (that is, squamous cell) carcinoma, the most common variety of vulvar cancer, is usually diagnosed at a less advanced stage than adenocarcinoma, which is a rare tumor that most often arises from Bartholin's glands. Epidermoid carcinoma tends to affect women who, on the average, are older than those affected by adenocarcinoma. Women who have epidermoid carcinoma of the vulva have been noted to have an increased incidence of epidermoid carcinoma of the cervix.

484. The answer is a. *(DiSaia, 5/e, pp 512–514.)* Alkylating agents (e.g., cyclophosphamide, chlorambucil, melphalan, thiotepa) act in all phases of the cell cycle; they cross-link the DNA. Hydroxyurea, doxorubicin, and methotrexate act primarily in the S phase (synthesis). Vincristine acts in the M phase (mitosis). Chemotherapy works by first-order kinetics; a certain percentage of cells are killed regardless of the number of actual tumor cells initially present. Kinetic studies suggest that tumors that have been cured by chemotherapy are those in which large fractions of cells are dividing (such as in gestational trophoblastic neoplasia). Bulky tumors (>2 cm) have longer generation times; this is the principle for tumor debulking in ovarian cancer.

485–486. The answers are 485-b,c,e; 486-a. *(Hoskins, 2/e, pp 78–79, 182, 197.)* Human papillomavirus (HPV) has been linked to cervical neoplasia, in particular types 16, 18, and 31. HPV types 6 and 11 are associated with benign condyloma. Two types of vulvar dystrophies exist: lichen sclerosus and hyperplastic dystrophy. When hyperplastic dystrophy is found to have atypical features, the lesion is thought to be premalignant. Lichen sclerosus is a benign condition that does not develop cellular atypia.

487–492. The answers are 487-b, 488-a, 489-a, 490-d, 491-c, 492-e. *(Griffiths, p 188.)* Sertoli-Leydig cell tumors, which represent less than 1% of ovarian tumors, may produce symptoms of virilization. Histologically, they resemble fetal testes; clinically, they must be distinguished from other functioning ovarian neoplasms as well as from tumors of the adrenal glands, since both adrenal tumors and Sertoli-Leydig tumors produce androgens. In turn, the androgen production can result in seborrhea, acne, menstrual irregularity, hirsutism, breast atrophy, alopecia, deepening of the voice, and clitoromegaly. Recurrences of Sertoli-Leydig cell tumors, which seem to have a low malignant potential, usually appear within 3 years of the original diagnosis. Granulosa and theca cell tumors are often associated with excessive estrogen production, which may cause pseudoprecocious puberty, postmenopausal bleeding, or menorrhagia. These tumors are associated with endometrial carcinoma in 15% of patients. Because these tumors are quite friable, affected women frequently present with symptoms caused by tumor rupture and intraperitoneal bleeding. Granulosa tumors are low-grade malignancies that tend to recur more than 5 years after the initial diagnosis. Because their malignant potential is impossible to predict histologically, long-term follow-up is mandatory. Recurrences have been reported as late as 33 years after the original diagnosis. Gonadoblastomas frequently contain calcifications that can be detected by plain radiography of the pelvis. Women who have gonadoblastomas often have ambiguous genitalia. The tumors are usually small and, in one-third of affected women, bilateral. The malignant potential of immature teratomas correlates with the degree of immature or embryonic tissue present. The presence of choriocarcinoma can be determined histologically as well as by human chorionic gonadotropin (hCG) assays. The presence of choriocarcinoma in an immature teratoma worsens the prognosis. Krukenberg tumors are typically bilateral, solid masses of the ovary that nearly always represent metastases from another organ, usually the stomach or large intestine. They contain large numbers of signet ring adenocarcinoma cells within a cellular hyperplastic but nonneoplastic ovarian stroma.

493–498. The answers are 493-a, 494-b, 495-j, 496-e, 497-h, 498-i. (*Hoskins, 2/e, pp 385–386, 393–394, 628–630.*) Cyclophosphamide is an alkylating agent that cross-links DNA and also inhibits DNA synthesis. Hemorrhagic cystitis and alopecia are common side effects. Cisplatin causes renal damage and neural toxicity. Patients must be well hydrated. Its mode of action does not fit a specific category. Taxol can produce allergic reactions and bone marrow depression. Bleomycin and doxorubicin are antibiotics whose side effects are pulmonary fibrosis and cardiac toxicity, respectively. Vincristine arrests cells in metaphase by binding microtubular proteins and preventing the formation of mitotic spindles. Peripheral neuropathy is a common side effect.

499–505. The answers are 499-f, 500-a, 501-g, 502-e, 503-c, 504-b, 505-d. (*Hoskins, 2/e, pp 4–9, 607–610.*) The tumor in question 499 is an opened mature cystic teratoma (dermoid tumor) in which hair is visible. The microscopic section in question 500 is a classical example of well-differentiated adenocarcinoma of the endometrium, showing cellular pleomorphism, nuclear atypia with mitoses, and back-to-back crowding of glands with obliteration of intervening stroma; the glandular architecture of the tissue is, however, maintained. Endometrial cancer is categorized by both stage and grade. The differentiation of a carcinoma is expressed as its grade. Grade I lesions are well differentiated; grade II lesions are moderately well differentiated; grade III lesions are poorly differentiated. An increasing grade—i.e., a decreasing degree of differentiation—implies worsening prognosis. Tumors may be of a mixed cell type—for example, squamous and adenocarcinoma—or may be mucinous, serous, or clear. Question 501 shows clear cell adenocarcinoma with large, pale staining cells. Clear cell carcinoma of the endometrium is similar to that arising in the cervix, vagina, and ovary, and the histologic appearance is similar in each of these organs. Diethylstilbestrol exposure has been associated with an increased incidence of vaginal and cervical clear cell carcinomas. The tumor's origins are suggested to be mesonephric duct remnants. The microscopic appearance of clear cell carcinoma is related to deposits of periodic acid–Schiff (PAS) stain–positive glycogen. These tumors characteristically occur in older women and are very aggressive. The section in question 502 shows mixed müllerian endometrial cancer. Mixed müllerian tumors refer to the combination of heterologous elements—that is, tissue of different sources (cartilage in this picture). Question 503 is an example of choriocarcinoma, showing sheets of malignant trophoblast. Malignant choriocarcinoma is a transformation of molar tissue or a de novo lesion arising from the placenta. There are significant degrees of cellular pleomorphism and anaplasia. Choriocarcinoma can be differentiated from invasive mole by the fact that the latter has chorionic villi and the former does not. Questions 504 and 505 show early- to mid-proliferative endometrium and late secretory endometrium, respectively. Proliferative and late secretory endometrium can be differentiated by the development of glandular tissue and secretory patterns. In question 504 the glands are just beginning to proliferate, and the section cuts through several coils as they course towards the surface epithelium on the left. In question 505 the glands are dilated and filled with amorphous (glycogen) material.

BIBLIOGRAPHY

ADASHI EY, ROCK JA, ROSENWAKS Z (EDS): *Reproductive Endocrinology, Surgery, and Technology,* vols 1 and 2. Philadelphia, Lippincott-Raven, 1996.

AMERICAN COLLEGE OF OBSTETRICIANS AND GYNECOLOGISTS, COMMITTEE ON ETHICS: Patient Choice: Maternal-Fetal Conflict (Committee Opinion No. 55), October 1987.

AVERY GB, FLETCHER MA, MACDONALD MG (EDS): *Neonatology: Pathophysiology and Management of the Newborn,* 5th ed. Philadelphia, Lippincott, Williams & Wilkins, 1999.

BENACERRAF BR (ED): *Ultrasound of Fetal Syndromes.* Philadelphia, Churchill Livingstone, 1998.

CUNNINGHAM FG, ET AL. (EDS): *Williams Obstetrics,* 20th ed. Stamford, CT, Appleton & Lange, 1997.

CURTIS MG, HOPKINS MP (EDS): *Glass's Office Gynecology,* 5th ed. Philadelphia, Lippincott, Williams & Wilkins, 1999.

DEWAN DM, HOOD DD (EDS): *Practical Obstetric Anesthesia.* Philadelphia, Saunders, 1997.

DISAIA PJ, CREASMAN WT (EDS): *Clinical Gynecologic Oncology,* 5th ed. St. Louis, Mosby, 1997.

FLEISHER AC, ET AL. (EDS): *Principles and Practice of Ultrasonography in Obstetrics and Gynecology,* 5th ed. Stamford, CT, Appleton & Lange, 1996.

GALL SA (ED): *Multiple Pregnancy and Delivery.* St. Louis, Mosby, 1996.

GIDWANI G, FALCONE T (EDS): *Congenital Malformations of the Female Genital Tract: Diagnosis and Management.* Philiadelphia, Lippincott, Williams & Wilkins, 1999.

GLEICHER N, ET AL. (EDS): *Principles and Practice of Medical Therapy in Pregnancy,* 3d ed. Stamford, CT, Appleton & Lange, 1998.

GRIFFITHS CT, SILVERSTONE A, TOBIAS J, BENAJMIN E (EDS.): *Gynecologic Oncology.* London, Mosby-Wolfe, 1997.

HANKINS GDV, ET AL. (EDS): *Operative Obstetrics.* Norwalk, CT, Appleton & Lange, 1995.

HEPPARD MCS, GARITE TJ (EDS): *Acute Obstetrics: A Practical Guide,* 2d ed. St. Louis, Mosby, 1996.

HOSKINS WJ, PEREZ CA, YOUNG RC (EDS): *Principles and Practice of Gynecologic Oncology,* 2d ed. Philadelphia, Lippincott, 1997.

JAFFE R, BUI TH (EDS): *Textbook of Fetal Ultrasonography.* London, Parthenon, 1999.

JAMES DK, ET AL. (EDS): *High Risk Pregnancy: Management Options,* 2d ed. London, Saunders, 1999.

JONES KL (ED): *Smith's Recognizable Patterns of Human Malformations,* 5th ed. Philadelphia, Saunders, 1997.

KEYE WR, ET AL. (EDS): *Infertility: Evaluation and Treatment.* Philadelphia, Saunders, 1995.

KORF BR (ED): *Human Genetics: A Problem-Based Approach.* Cambridge, MA, Blackwell Science, 1996.

LAMBROU NC, MORSE AN, WALLACH EE (EDS): *The Johns Hopkins Manual of Gynecology and Obstetrics.* Baltimore, Lippincott, Williams & Wilkins, 1999.

LOBO RA (ED): *Treatment of the Postmenopausal Woman,* 2d ed. Philadelphia, Lippincott, Williams & Wilkins, 1999.

MISHELL DR, STENCHEVER MA, DROEGENMUELLER W, HERBST AL (EDS): *Comprehensive Gynecology,* 3d ed. St. Louis, Mosby, 1997.

QUEENAN JT (ED): *Management of High Risk Pregnancy,* 4th ed. Malden, MA, Blackwell Science, 1999.

RANSOM SB, DOMBROWSKI MP, MCNEELEY SG, MOGHISSI K, MUNKARAH AR (EDS): *Practical Strategies in Obstetrics and Gynecology.* Philadelphia, Saunders, 2000.

RANSOM SB, MCNEELEY SG (EDS): *Gynecology for the Primary Care Provider.* Philadelphia, Saunders, 1997.

REECE EA, ET AL. (EDS): *Medicine of the Fetus and Mother,* 2d ed. Philadelphia, Lippincott, 1999.

REMOIN RL, CONNOR JM, PYERITZ RE (EDS): *Principles and Practice of Medical Genetics,* 3d ed. New York, Churchill Livingstone, 1996.

ROCK JA, THOMPSON JD (EDS): *TeLinde's Operative Gynecology,* 8th ed. Philadelphia, Lippincott-Raven, 1997.

RODECK CH, WHITTLE MJ (EDS): *Fetal Medicine: Basic Science and Clinical Practice.* London, Churchill Livingstone, 1999.

SCHWARTZ SI, SHIRES GT, SPENCER FC (EDS): *Principles of Surgery,* 7th ed. New York, McGraw-Hill, 1999.

SCOTT JR, ET AL. (EDS): *Danforth's Obstetrics and Gynecology,* 8th ed. Philadelphia, Lippincott-Raven, 1999.

Speroff L, Glass RH, Kase NG (eds): *Clinical Gynecologic Endocrinology and Infertility,* 6th ed. Baltimore, Lippincott, Williams & Wilkins, 1999.

Timor-Tritsch JE, Monteagudo A, Cohen HL (eds): *Ultrasonography of the Prenatal and Neonatal Brain.* Stamford, CT, Appleton & Lange, 1996.

Zatuchni GI, Slupik RI: *Obstetrics and Gynecology Drug Handbook,* St. Louis, Mosby, 1996.

ISBN 0-07-135961-3

90000

9 780071 359610